BRIEF ALCOHOL SCREENING AND INTERVENTION FOR COLLEGE STUDENTS (BASICS)

BRIEF ALCOHOL SCREENING AND INTERVENTION FOR COLLEGE STUDENTS (BASICS)

A Harm Reduction Approach

Linda A. Dimeff
John S. Baer
Daniel R. Kivlahan
G. Alan Marlatt

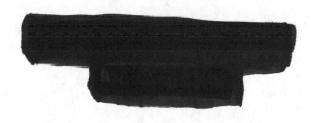

THE GUILFORD PRESS
New York   London

© 1999 The Guilford Press
A Division of Guilford Publications, Inc.
72 Spring Street, New York, NY 10012
http://www.guilford.com

Printed in the United States of America.

This book is printed on acid-free paper.

Last digit is print number: 9 8 7 6 5 4 3 2 1

Library of Congress Cataloging-in-Publication Data

Brief Alcohol Screening and Intervention for College Students (BASICS)
 : a harm reduction approach / Linda A. Dimeff . . . [et a
   p.   cm.
  Includes bibliographical references and index.
  ISBN 1-57230-392-1
   1. College students—Alcohol use. 2. Alcoholism—Prevention.
 3. Alcoholism—Study and teaching. 4. College students—Counseling of.
 I. Dimeff, Linda A.
 [DNLM: 1. Alcohol Drinking—prevention and control. 2. Student Health
 Services—methods. 3. Alcoholism—prevention and control. 4. Students—
 psychology. 5. Counseling—methods. 6. Cognitive Therapy—methods.
 WA 353 B853 1998]
 HV5135.B74   1998
 362.292'7'0842—dc21
 DNLM/DLC
 for Library of Congress   98-46593
                                                              CIP

*To those who have experienced first-hand
the devastation wrought by alcohol misuse.*

About the Authors

Linda A. Dimeff, PhD, is a Research Scientist in the Department of Psychology at the University of Washington. Her research and clinical interests range from prevention of alcohol problems in college students to treatment of severely disordered substance abusing individuals with borderline personality disorder. Funded by two grant awards, her dissertation was a replication and extension of BASICS applied in a student health center setting and using multimedia computers, along with provider advice.

John S. Baer, PhD, is Research Associate Professor of Psychology at the University of Washington, and is currently Coordinator of Education at the National Center of Excellence for Substance Abuse Treatment and Education at the VA Puget Sound Health Care System. Dr. Baer's research and clinical interests focus on the assessment, early intervention, and relapse of substance use and abuse. He is the recipient of local and national research grants examining secondary prevention and etiology of alcohol problems.

Daniel R. Kivlahan, PhD, is Director of the National Center of Excellence in Substance Abuse Treatment and Education at the VA Puget Sound Health Care System and Associate Professor of Psychiatry and Behavioral Sciences at the University of Washington School of Medicine. He continues to pursue health services research related to substance use disorders, including development, implementation, and evaluation of evidence-based clinical practice guidelines.

G. Alan Marlatt, PhD, is currently Professor of Psychology and Director of the Addictive Behaviors Research Center at the University of Washington. His major focus in both research and clinical work is the field of additive behaviors. In 1990, Dr. Marlatt was awarded The Jellinek Memorial Award for outstanding contributions to knowledge in the field of alcohol studies. In 1996, he was appointed as a member of the National Advisory Council on Drug Abuse for the National Institute on Drug Abuse (NIH).

Acknowledgments

The work described in this book was built on the efforts of many individuals at the Addictive Behaviors Research Center (ABRC) at the University of Washington over the past several years. We are indebted to each of them for their intellectual contributions, which led to the development and refinement of BASICS. In particular, we wish to thank Kim Fromme, PhD, Mary Larimer, PhD, Ellen Williams, Martin Stern, PhD, Julian Somers, PhD, and Lori Quigley, PhD. Each of these individuals contributed in a variety of invaluable ways, from wrangling with the research design in our original grant submission to stuffing participant recruitment packets, analyzing data, interviewing students, and critiquing this intervention. Kim Barret, EdD, and George Parks, PhD, served as research therapists on this project and also provided incisive clinical insights which helped mold this intervention. We thank Jason Kilmer, PhD, and Eleanor Kim, PhD, for their creativity in implementing BASICS and the Alcohol Skills Training Program in all kinds of settings and for their unique capacity to engage student audiences. We are indebted to Lorraine Collins, PhD, for urging us to think about gender differences in risks associated with alcohol consumption during her stay at the ABRC as a visiting scholar.

Many people provided much-needed administrative support as we implemented various phases of this project. A special thanks to Sally Weatherford, PhD, our administrator and colleague, for her extensive work in mobilizing the assistance we needed to complete this manuscript for its submission, which included spending numerous hours reformatting the text. We are also grateful to her and Ellen Williams for their tireless dedication to keeping our laboratory running smoothly and efficiently. We thank Jewel Brien, our original data manager and graphic artist, for her creative design of our forms and personalized feedback materials. Thanks to Susan Tapert, PhD, Dan Irvine, and Rebekka Palmer for their administrative support and gathering materials needed for publication. Eugene Isyanov and Frank Provo spent many hours editing the manuscript, locating references, and generating graphics. John Tucker pitched in at the last minute to generate a series of additional and much needed graphics.

We owe the staff at The Guilford Press a debt of gratitude for their help in bringing this book to fruition. We wish to specifically thank our editors, Rochelle Serwator and Jeannie Tang, for identifying the value of this project and moving it along to completion; Marie Sprayberry for her outstanding copyediting; and William Meyer and Paul Gordon for their enormous patience and their work on the graphics and artwork.

The research behind BASICS would not have come about but for the generous support of the National Institute on Alcohol and Alcoholism (NIAAA) at the National Institute of Health, which provided funding through a MERIT award and a Research Scientist award.

Finally, we are grateful to the hundreds of college students who have participated in our research over the years. They provided us with invaluable feedback about their experiences involving alcohol use and suggestions for how we could further strengthen and refine our programs.

Contents

BRIEF ALCOHOL SCREENING AND INTERVENTION FOR COLLEGE STUDENTS (BASICS)

Introduction

Many college administrators, counselors, and student health primary care providers are well aware of the problems associated with alcohol abuse in college students; they are determined to find effective policies and programs to prevent or reduce alcohol consumption, in addition to decreasing alcohol-related problems. The task of preventing alcohol abuse in college students is by no means an easy one, as anyone who has attempted interventions for this widespread problem knows. Currents running counter to preventive efforts include the age-specific developmental challenges many young people face as they leave home for the first time and begin experimenting with many adult behaviors, including sexual intimacy and alcohol use. Complicating matters further is the fact that young adults are subjected to a barrage of powerful messages from alcohol advertisements that prey on their vulnerability and youth. What could be more important for many young adults, for example, than fitting in socially with their peers and being perceived by others as sexually attractive (the message conveyed by many beer and wine commercials)?

Efforts to prevent alcohol problems in college students can take many different forms and can target very different audiences at various levels of involvement with drinking alcohol—from delaying the first drink in abstainers, to preventing more serious problems from occurring in students who already drink heavily and may be experiencing at least minimal problems as a result. The specific prevention program described in this manual is designed for the latter group: individual students who already drink heavily and have experienced, or are at high risk of experiencing, alcohol-related problems. This type of prevention is referred to as **indicated prevention** (formally, as **secondary prevention**), because of its focus on high-risk students who may already be developing slight yet detectable evidence of the problem (Gordon, 1987; Institute of Medicine, 1995). Indicated prevention programs are obviously different from programs that are directed at all college students (**universal prevention**), or from programs targeting subgroups of college students who are at risk for alcohol abuse because of unique personal characteristics or lifestyle associated with alcohol abuse (e.g., a history of conduct disorder, membership in a fraternity or sorority), but who either have not yet initiated drinking or have not yet begun to drink heavily (**selective prevention**).

Along with our colleagues at the University of Washington's Addictive Behaviors Research Center, we have spent well over 15 years developing and testing the efficacy of several indicated prevention programs, with the majority of our research participants in these studies meeting DSM-III-R and DSM-IV diagnostic criteria for alcohol abuse (American Psychiatric Association, 1987, 1994). The present manual focuses exclusively on one of these programs: the Brief Alcohol Screening and Intervention for College Students (BASICS), a two-session brief intervention. In comparison to a control group of students who completed annual assessments only, students receiving BASICS reported statistically significant reductions in their use of alcohol and reported experiencing significantly fewer negative consequences resulting from alcohol (Marlatt et al., in press).

While incorporating a number of state-of-the-art components for brief interventions (Heather, 1995), BASICS was designed specifically for college students who abuse alcohol. BASICS is based on a model that combines capability deficits, as well as developmental and motivational aspects. This model assumes that (1) many of these students lack important information and coping skills to drink moderately; (2) certain developmental milestones contribute to heavy drinking (e.g., separation from parents and assumption of adult activities); and (3) personal factors (e.g., faulty beliefs about alcohol) and environmental factors (e.g., peer pressure, heavy-drinking friends, cultural mindset of "drink until drunk") inhibit the use of behavioral skills that the students have in their repertoires.

BASICS uses a harm reduction approach. That is, its primary goal is to move a student in the direction of reducing risky behaviors and harmful effects from drinking as opposed to focusing explicitly on a specific drinking goal (e.g., abstinence or reductions in drinking). In a nutshell, harm reduction is a continuum model for change. Recognizing that lifestyle changes usually occur gradually over time, practitioners of harm reduction emphasize and encourage incremental changes (e.g., proximal goals over distal goals), and they view steps in the direction of reducing harmful or hazardous behavior as success. These principles are not unlike the basic behavioral principles of shaping, in which a therapist reinforces successive approximations of the new behavior. The spirit of harm reduction, however, encompasses more than a mechanical approach to change. Assumptions that are rooted in harm reduction and that inform our development of BASICS and our approach with college drinkers include the following (Beadnell, Baker, Gordon, Roffman, & Carver, 1995):

- Student-chosen drinking goals are more powerful than drinking goals articulated or required by others.

- The factors that maintain heavy drinking in college students are different from those factors that maintain heavy drinking in older adults; a brief intervention for college students is most likely to be effective if it addresses these unique factors.

- Risk reduction, without further specification of outcomes (e.g., abstinence, full moderation from drinking), is itself a valid goal for a brief intervention for high-risk drinkers.

- The goals of a brief intervention focused on college students should be realistic and achievable, even if they don't eliminate all risks.

- Behavioral "slips" are normal.

- Moderate drinking to decrease harmful effects can be as enjoyable as heavy, hazardous drinking.

- Successful experiences in the direction of achieving goals are more important than immediate and complete elimination of risk.

- Risk reduction can continue indefinitely, with students continuing to practice and improve over time.

- The least intensive intervention should be applied first before proceeding to more intensive interventions (stepped-care approach).

FOR WHOM IS THIS MANUAL DESIGNED?

This manual is designed as a self-contained workbook for those providing prevention, education, and treatment services to college students who drink alcohol. Therapists need not have a great deal of knowledge about alcohol or extensive specialized training in addictions counseling to understand and make use of the contents of this manual. Nevertheless, we have found it important for users of this manual to have a familiarity with basic counseling skills.

BASICS is intended for heavy-drinking college undergraduates who either have experienced problems because of heavy consumption or are at high risk of doing so. Many students receiving this brief intervention meet DSM-IV criteria for alcohol abuse or mild alcohol dependence. **Alcohol abuse** is defined as the continued use of alcohol despite problems that are clearly caused or exacerbated by alcohol use, or continued use of alcohol while engaging in activities that could be dangerous when a person is intoxicated (e.g., driving while intoxicated, attending to children, etc.). Alcohol abuse is essentially a pattern of drinking that has resulted in detrimental health effects, social difficulties, and/or legal problems. **Alcohol dependence** is characterized by excessive alcohol-seeking behaviors that lead to impaired control over alcohol use and often includes the physiological changes of tolerance and withdrawal. The DSM-IV criteria for substance abuse and substance dependence (these apply to all classes of substances; separate criteria sets for alcohol abuse and alcohol dependence are not provided) are reprinted in Table I.1. BASICS is not intended for students with moderate to severe alcohol dependence.

TABLE I.1. DSM-IV Criteria for Substance Abuse and Substance Dependence

Substance Abuse

A. A maladaptive pattern of substance use, leading to clinically significant impairment or distress, as manifested by one (or more) of the following, occurring within a 12-month period:

   (1) recurrent substance use resulting in a failure to fulfill major obligations at work, school, or home (e.g., repeated absences or poor work performance related to substance use; substance-related absences, suspensions, or expulsions from school; neglect of children or household)

   (2) recurrent substance use in situations in which it is physically hazardous (e.g., driving an automobile or operating a machine when impaired by substance use)

   (3) recurrent substance-related legal problems (e.g., arrests for substance-related disorderly conduct)

   (4) continued substance use despite having persistent or recurrent social or interpersonal problems caused or exacerbated by the effects of the substance (e.g., arguments with spouse about consequences of intoxication, physical fights)

B. The symptoms have never met the criteria for Substance Dependence for this class of substance.

Substance Dependence

A maladaptive pattern of substance use, leading to clinically significant impairment or distress, as manifested by three (or more) of the following, occurring at any time in the same 12-month period:

(1) tolerance, as defined by either of the following:

   (a) a need for markedly increased amounts of the substance to achieve intoxication or desired effect

   (b) markedly diminished effect with continued use of the same amount of the substance

(2) withdrawal, as manifested by either of the following:

   (a) the characteristic withdrawal syndrome for the substance (refer to Criteria A and B of the criteria sets for Withdrawal from the specific substances)

   (b) the same (or a closely related) substance is taken to relieve or avoid withdrawal symptoms

(3) the substance is often taken in larger amounts or over a longer period than was intended.

(4) there is a persistent desire or unsuccessful efforts to cut down or control substance use

(5) a great deal of time is spent in activities necessary to obtain the substance (e.g., driving long distances), use the substance (e.g., chain smoking) or recover from its effects

(6) important social, occupational, or recreational activities are given up or reduced because of substance use

(7) the substance use is continued despite knowledge of having a persistent or recurrent physical or psychological problem that is likely to have been caused or exacerbated by the substance (e.g., continued drinking despite recognition that an ulcer was made worse by alcohol consumption)

(continued)

BASICS IN A NUTSHELL

Our Alcohol Skills Training Program (ASTP) is a skills-based curriculum that aims to reduce harmful consumption and associated problems in students who drink alcohol. The ASTP approach provides specific cognitive-behavioral strategies for moderate, lower-risk drinking. BASICS is one of several intervention modalities that fall under the general umbrella of ASTP. Of all the modalities, BASICS is the least intensive and

TABLE I-1. *continued*

Specify if:

With Physiological Dependence: evidence of tolerance or withdrawal (i.e., either Item 1 or 2 is present)

Without Physiological Dependence: no evidence of tolerance or withdrawal (i.e., either Item 1 nor 2 is present)

Course specifiers (see text for definitions):

Early Full Remission

Early Partial Remission

Sustained Full Remission

Sustained Partial Remission

On Agonist Therapy

In a Controlled Environment

Note. Reprinted with permission from the *Diagnostic and Statistical Manual of Mental Disorders, Fourth Edition.* Copyright 1994 by the American Psychiatric Association.

the most flexible and personalized. BASICS is nonconfrontational, nonjudgmental, nonauthoritarian, and nonlabeling.

BASICS is conducted over the course of two 50-minute interview sessions (with an additional 50 minutes allowed before or after the first interview for the student to complete self-report questionnaires). In the first interview, the therapist assesses the student's consumption pattern and apprises the student of negative behavioral consequences stemming from use of alcohol and other behaviors that may contribute to the student's health risks. Personalized feedback based on the assessment, and specific advice about ways to reduce future health risks associated with alcohol use, are then reviewed in the subsequent meeting. Consistent with the literature on brief interventions, our own research has demonstrated that two meetings are generally sufficient for students to make substantial changes in their drinking patterns and to reduce negative consequences of alcohol use. In some cases, BASICS may be the first step toward seeking additional services to initiate or maintain changes. Additional services can range in intensity from a single booster session of BASICS to more traditional outpatient or inpatient treatment.

The BASICS techniques and therapeutic approach described in this manual may have broader applications beyond the one-to-one interaction between therapist and student described herein. One logical extension is to apply these same procedures to small groups of students who are seeking services for alcohol-related problems. The same or similar procedures could also be applied to larger social groups with strong community identities and established drinking norms (e.g., sororities and fraternities, athletic teams). In the latter case, the collective group, team, or house would serve as the unit of treatment, rather than the distinct individuals within the group. Moreover, BASICS may be an effective indicated preventive intervention within college student primary health care facilities; in this setting, it would augment preventive health care provided to students who drink. Several studies that build upon the initial brief intervention described in this manual are currently underway at the University of Washington.

HOW TO USE THIS MANUAL

BASICS was initially designed to reduce alcohol consumption and related problems in college students. The assessment described in this manual provides a basis for talking with students about their pattern of alcohol consumption and potential health risks associated with their level of use, as well as specific strategies to assist in reducing these risks. Although heavy consumption of alcohol among college students constitutes a significant public health matter, it is by no means the only risky behavior posing health concerns for this population. In the event that other risky or problematic health behaviors are presented (e.g., unsafe sex, disordered eating, abuse of other substances, etc.), readers are encouraged to tailor this brief intervention to the needs of their clients by broadening the range of health behaviors assessed and addressed.

We recognize that not all schools and programs wishing to implement BASICS will be able to do so in the manner we describe in this manual. A number of college administrators and care providers have commented, for example, that they simply lack the resources and time to meet with students on more than one occasion. This manual describes the exact protocol we used for our empirical test of BASICS' efficacy. It is often the case in research studies that lengthy questionnaires with sound psychometric properties are required to measure and document the findings reliably. For example, while one set of drinking measures may have been sufficient to assess students' patterns of alcohol consumption, we included various other measures to adhere to the rigors of research. Naturally, what is required for research is not necessarily required for good clinical work. We hope to dismantle the components of BASICS to pinpoint the most robust aspects of the intervention. In the meantime, we offer some suggestions of what we believe is essential to include, based on our clinical experience and research.

Although readers may benefit considerably from reading other sources cited in this manual, no additional reading is necessary in order to apply the manual's basic contents. We have attempted to provide sufficient coverage of pertinent conceptual and clinical material—that is, to provide both a theoretical foundation and specific instructions in how to operationalize BASICS. A conceptual and epidemiological overview of college drinking is provided in Chapter 1. A description of ASTP is given in Chapter 2. Chapter 3 lays the foundation for BASICS; it includes descriptions of theoretical approaches to preventing harm from alcohol use, basic information about alcohol, and the BASICS format and clinical aims. Chapters 4 and 5 describe the two sessions of BASICS—the initial assessment interview and the feedback interview, respectively. Chapter 6 discusses various clinical concerns and pitfalls that are commonly encountered during the implementation of BASICS. Four appendices discuss relevant assessment instruments; provide examples of personalized graphic feedback and "tips" sheets; furnish other informational handouts for students; and present a selection of published and unpublished assessment measures.

CHAPTER 1

Alcohol Use and Prevention of Alcohol Abuse in College Students

Our primary objective in this chapter is to provide a theoretical and empirical overview of issues pertinent to addressing alcohol problems among college students. We review patterns of alcohol use and its consequences among college students; possible prevention approaches with this population; risk factors associated with alcohol use in college students; barriers to effective prevention and treatment for underage drinkers; and recommendations for prevention and treatment by the Institute of Medicine (1990) and others.

PATTERNS OF ALCOHOL USE AND CONSEQUENCES AMONG COLLEGE STUDENTS

Despite decades of prevention efforts and public health policies, heavy and hazardous drinking among college students (especially undergraduates) remains a formidable and vexing public health concern. In two nationwide surveys of college students, nearly 85% of undergraduates reported drinking alcohol in the past year (Johnston, O'Malley, & Bachman, 1996; Presley, Meilman, & Lyerla, 1995). In one of these surveys, 62.5% of college students reported using alcohol in the past 30 days; 3.6% reported daily use (Johnston et al., 1996). In the other survey, which included over 45,000 students from 87 U.S. undergraduate institutions, 19.2% of the sample reported using alcohol on at least three occasions weekly (27.3% of men and 13.9% of women; Presley et al., 1995).

In addition to the widespread prevalence of alcohol use by college students and the frequency with which they consume alcohol, many students drink in a heavy, hazardous fashion. In the comprehensive survey by Presley et al. (1995), college students reported consuming an average of 4.3 drinks per week (6.7 drinks for men, 3.0 drinks for women); 10% of these students consumed 15 or more drinks on an average weekly basis (Meilman, Presley, & Cashin, 1997). Wechsler Davenport, Dowdall, and Moeykens (1994) surveyed 17,592 students at 140 colleges and found that 44% engaged in **binge drinking,** defined as five or more drinks in a row for men and four drinks in a row for women on at least one occasion in the 2 weeks prior to completing the survey. Nineteen percent of this sample reported frequent episodes of binge drinking (three or more binge episodes in the preceding 2 weeks). Engs, Diebold, and Hanson (1996) surveyed 12,000 from every state in the United States during the 1993–1994 academic year and identified 20.6% as heavy drinkers (consuming 5 or more drinks per occasion on at least a weekly basis). While the average student consumed 9.6 drinks weekly, 31% of the men typically consumed over 21 drinks weekly and 19.2% of the women typically consumed over 14 drinks weekly.

Drinking among college students fluctuates considerably throughout the academic year and is typically tied to major events (e.g., homecoming games and completion of finals) and to academic breaks. Smeaton, Josiam, and Dietrich (1998) recently surveyed a convenience sample of 442 women and 341 men vacationing during their academic spring break at Panama City Beach, Florida. On average, men reported consuming 18 drinks and women reported consuming 10 drinks on the preceding day; additionally, 91.7% of the men and 78.1% of the women reported at least one episode of binge drinking during the preceding day. Although these data are startling, heavy alcohol consumption among college students in the United States has a long and well-documented history (Berkowitz & Perkins, 1986; Brennan, Walfish, & AuBuchon, 1986; Saltz & Elandt, 1986; Straus & Bacon, 1953).

Results from a random survey of 1,595 students conducted at the University of Washington (Lowell, 1993) provide further evidence to illustrate the extent to which undergraduates in particular are at risk for alcohol problems. The University of Washington is a large academic institution located in Seattle that provides undergraduate- and graduate-level training to over 35,000 students. More than half the students who participated in the survey were light drinkers or nondrinkers, but undergraduates tended to drink in a more excessive fashion than graduate students did. Although more undergraduates than graduate students abstained from drinking (28.6% and 19.0%, respectively), nearly twice as many undergraduates as graduate students reported binge drinking (31% and 17%, respectively).

Consumption of alcohol remains implicated in nearly all behavioral and health problems experienced by young adults, including sexual aggression (Norris, Nurius, & Dimeff, 1996; Koss, Gidycz, & Wisniewski, 1987), impaired academic performance (Wood, Sher, Erickson, & DeBord, 1997; Presley et al., 1995), vandalism and fighting (Engs et al., 1996; Engs, Engs, & Hanson, 1990, 1985), sexually transmitted diseases (Donovan & McEwan, 1995; Strunin & Hingson, 1992) and motor vehicle accidents and fatalities (Campbell, Zobeck, & Bertolucci, 1995; National Highway Traffic Safety Administration, 1994). In a survey study of college administrators, alcohol use was directly linked to residence hall damage (67%), violent behaviors (65%), and student attrition (29%) (Anderson & Gadaleto, 1994). Alcohol involvement was suspected nearly half the time in property damage incidents (47%), injuries to other people (46%), self-injuries (43%), and lowered academic performance (41%) (Anderson & Presley, 1991). Recent reports of "secondhand" effects of alcohol use have appeared in the research literature, providing further documentation of the far-reaching effects of heavy drinking on other members of the campus community. In another study, 43% of those surveyed reported disruptions in study or sleep habits; 21% reported experiencing unwanted sexual advances; and 27% described being humiliated or insulted by someone who had been drinking (Wechsler, Moeykens, Bavenport, Castillo, & Hansen, 1995).

As one might expect, harmful consequences of drinking rise in proportion to the amount of alcohol consumed (O'Hare, 1990). Results from the survey by Presley et al. (1995) reveal an association between heavy drinking and poor scholastic achievement, with "A" students reporting an average of 3.2 drinks consumed weekly in comparison to "D" students, who reportedly consumed 8.4 drinks on average. Wechsler, Davenport et al. (1994) reported that nearly half of frequent binge drinkers were 7 to 10 times more likely than those who were not binge drinkers to engage in unplanned sexual activity and/or unprotected sexual intercourse, to get hurt or injured, to get into trouble with campus or local police, to damage property, and to drive after having five or more drinks.

Importantly, adolescent and young adult drinking patterns are neither fixed nor static, but change considerably over time (Grant, Harford, & Grigoon, 1988). Among those who attend college, drinking rates increase substantially in the transition from high school to the freshman year (Baer, Kivlahan, & Marlatt, 1995); the rates then decrease steadily after the first year (Marlatt et al., 1998a; Zucker & Fitzgerald, 1991; Jessor, Donovan, & Costa, 1991), possibly as students mature and assume additional "adult" responsibilities. Epidemiologist Kaye Fillmore (1988) observed that young adults are at greatest risk for alcohol problems during their early 20s, with two-thirds of problem drinkers "maturing out" of heavy drinking patterns without treatment by their late 20s.

PREVENTION APPROACHES FOR COLLEGE STUDENTS

Although the vast majority of college students will outgrow heavy drinking and alcohol-related problems without assistance or treatment, they are nonetheless vulnerable to a myriad of harmful consequences until they do so. Therefore, a reasonable objective for prevention programming may be to help students move safely through this risky developmental period. How best to accomplish this objective is largely speculative, however. Some college health administrators are advocating for comprehensive, campus-wide interventions that involve managing the campus environment (e.g., making campus a drug-free zone, sponsoring alcohol-free parties and other activities as alternatives to drinking) and integrating alcohol education and prevention efforts into existing campus-based activities (e.g., incorporating lectures on alcohol and potential problems into courses). Others also recommend inoculating individuals against harm by providing the necessary skills to keep safe within a party context and the motivation to use them (Marlatt et al., 1998).

As we have noted earlier, efforts at preventing alcohol-related problems in college students can target very different audiences at very different drinking levels. Gordon (1987) classifies three types of preventive interventions—**universal, indicated,** and **selective**—on the basis of an individual's risk for developing a particular problem and the cost of the intervention (see also Institute of Medicine, 1995). Universal prevention efforts are directed at all members of a population (in this case, all undergraduates at a college or university). Indicated prevention measures are directed at individuals who are already experiencing at least some manifestations of a particular problem, or who possess risk factors identified statistically as greatly increasing the probability of a particular problem in the future (e.g., current heavy use of alcohol predicts continued heavy use). Finally, selected prevention measures target members of a subgroup known to be at risk for developing a problem. In the case of college students, such subgroups include sorority or fraternity members (Larimer, 1992), first-year students (Baer et al., 1995), members of an athletic team (Tricker & Cook, 1989), and persons with a history of conduct disorder (King, Ghaziuddin, McGovern, & Brand, 1996).

Efforts in all three prevention categories to reduce heavy and hazardous drinking on college campuses have mushroomed over the past decade. In a recent comprehensive review of 811 alcohol prevention programs on colleges and universities across the United States, Anderson and Milgram (1996) found that 98% of respondents reported having a specific site designated for resource materials; that 74% reported having a designated alcohol/substance abuse coordinator or specialist (in comparison to 14% in 1979); that 60% offered an undergraduate course that included materials on alcohol abuse; that 90% designated "alcohol awareness" days or weeks; and that 59% offered support groups on campus.

It is also important to consider the level or intensity of an intervention, especially when it is directed at an individual (Keller, Bennett, McCrady, Paulus, & Frankenstein, 1994). One approach is to match the intensity of the intervention with the severity and chronicity of the problem. That is, individuals with brief histories of alcohol use and mild to moderate problems are first provided a minimal intervention, with the degree of intensity of the intervention increasing as necessary until the necessary therapeutic impact is achieved. This sequential, stepped approach is consistent with the Institute of Medicine's (1990) recommendation for broadening the base of treatment to include prevention efforts for persons (e.g., college students) who are at risk for alcohol problems but may never develop alcohol dependence or experience moderate to severe levels of alcohol-related problems.

RISK FACTORS ASSOCIATED WITH COLLEGE DRINKING

Factors associated with the initiation of drinking, regular use of alcohol, and abuse of alcohol in young adults involve complex developmental processes, environmental influences, and individual differences in response to alcohol. Moreover, the factors associated with the initiation of use often differ from those associated with continued use or development of problems. Research that examines how risk factors combine to create a risk profile is much needed. An individual's risk may increase in an additive or a multiplicative fashion (Bry, McKeon, & Pandina, 1982). Zucker, Fitzgerald, and Moses (1995) suggest that an individual's risk for alcohol problems is probably based on the extent to which a preexisting structure of risky biology interacts with and is exacerbated by the environmental context.

Peer influence is the most common environmental risk factor for alcohol use in adolescence and is the single best predictor of young adult drinking (Jessor & Jessor, 1977; Kandel & Andrews, 1987). Peers are commonly believed to "socialize" one another to drink by modeling, imitating, or reinforcing drinking behavior. Interestingly, in addition to the socializing effect, peer influence seems to interact with a "peer selection" process. Numerous studies have shown, for example, that persons choose to associate with peers who are similar to themselves and whose lifestyle resembles theirs (Jacob & Leonard, 1991; Kandel, 1986). Environmental factors such as residence (Larimer, 1992) and "party" setting (Geller & Kalsher, 1990; Geller, Russ, & Altomari, 1986) also contribute to risk. Findings from our own research show that students who are already drinking heavily while in high school select college living arrangements where heavy drinking is a social norm (e.g., fraternities) (Baer et al., 1995). Once the students are living in this environment, their drinking increases still further. One outcome of this socialization/selection process is that students often perceive their drinking as falling well within the typical range of college student consumption, even when it is well above the average (Baer, Stacy, & Larimer, 1991).

Personal dispositional factors, such as a family history of alcoholism (Sher, Walitzer, Wood, & Brent, 1991), may also contribute to risk of developing alcohol problems. Adult studies have shown that a genetic history of alcohol problems may increase an individual's risk for alcohol problems (Sher et al., 1991), even when the child is reared by adoptive parents (Cadoret, 1990). Other studies find that drinking behavior is negatively reinforced in adolescents whose parents drink excessively (Harburg, Davis, & Caplan, 1982). Although the offspring of abstinent parents are more likely to abstain themselves, they are more likely to drink in a deviant fashion when they do drink (Barnes, Farrell, & Cairns, 1986). Other dispositional factors include a history of an acting-out personality style or conduct-disordered behavior, characterized by sensation seeking, impulsivity, and inability to delay gratification (Jessor, 1991). In their research on adolescent behavior, Jessor and Jessor (1977) coined the term **problem behavior syndrome** to describe the pattern in which many young people who drink early and with greater frequency are also likely to have difficulties with truancy, other drug use, and precocious sexual activity.

Differences in social environment and individual responses to alcohol lead to different expectations and beliefs about the effects of alcohol. Positive alcohol outcome expectancies, false beliefs, and misattributions about alcohol are related to heavy consumption and high risks (Mooney, Fromme, Kivlahan, & Marlatt, 1987; Stacy, Widaman, & Marlatt, 1990). Marlatt and other researchers (Fromme, Kivlahan, & Marlatt, 1986; Southwick, Steele, Marlatt, & Lindell, 1981; Christensen, Goldman, & Brown, 1985; Brown, Christensen, & Goldman, 1987; Leigh, 1987, 1989) have found that positive alcohol outcome expectancies are positively correlated with heavy consumption. Expectancies found to be highly correlated with consumption include increased self-confidence, sociability, social disinhibition, and physical/sexual attractiveness. Particularly for a group of young adults, many of whom are relatively new to dating and engaging in sexual relations, the perceived benefit of alcohol are obviously seductive and rewarding. In a recent study of alcohol-related expectancies among 367 college fraternity and sorority members, the strongest predictor of heavy drinking was the belief that alcohol makes it easier to act out sexually (Larimer, Irvine, Kilmer, & Marlatt, 1997). A male student attending our center recently remarked, "I was at a party the other night and saw this woman across the room that I really liked. I would have never had the nerve to meet her if I hadn't been pounding drinks." In this sense, alcohol is perceived to serve as a social lubricant by enhancing an individual's sense of self-adequacy, while also providing an excuse for and/or an outlet for social disinhibition.

In addition to their positive alcohol expectancies, many college students, particularly those who are less experienced drinkers, commonly believe that the degree of enjoyment derived from alcohol is directly related to the amount consumed. This false belief about alcohol is captured by the saying, "If some is good, more is better." As drinkers become more experienced, they generally reach a **"point of diminishing return"**—that is, a point at which another drink no longer enhances enjoyment but may instead increase discomfort and minimize enjoyment. We have frequently been told by older students that they used to drink heavily when they were freshmen and sophomores, but now "it's no longer fun to get smashed the way we used to." Often through experience, students will purposely alter their drinking habits to avoid negative effects of heavy alcohol use (e.g., hangovers and embarrassment). Unfortunately, younger students or inexperienced drinkers continue to fall prey to the "more is better" belief, which can promote heavy drinking.

Last but by no means least, developmental issues contribute to heavy alcohol consumption (Shedler & Block, 1990). Experimenting with alcohol and other drugs, and experiencing altered states of consciousness, are common rites of passage into adulthood and autonomy in modern Western culture. For many young adults, college provides a first opportunity to act like an older adult. Alcohol can be obtained easily (even by underage students) and consumed openly. In addition, many see their college years as their last opportunity to "cut loose" before setting foot into the realities of postgraduation adulthood and professional careers. A student recently referred to our center for violation of a university alcohol policy commented, "Once I graduate, my drinking habits will change. I'll have a real job and responsibilities, and I won't be able to party all the time."

BARRIERS TO EFFECTIVE PREVENTION AND TREATMENT

Despite the increased concern about and attention to addressing heavy drinking on college campuses, a number of barriers have served to compromise the development and implementation of effective programming for undergraduates who choose to drink. Barriers typically fall into one of three categories: programmatic/institutional, personal, or conceptual.

Programmatic/Institutional Barriers

One common barrier to effective alcohol programming is the view that providing information about alcohol or harm reduction messages about moderation to underage students is equivalent to granting these students permission to drink. The dilemma we face is how to address the problem of heavy drinking and its consequences, while acknowledging the illegality of alcohol use for those under the statutory drinking age. Some may fear that by not addressing the illegality of this behavior through abstinence-only programming, we send the message that it is "okay" to break the law. Others may have less concern about breaking the law, and more concern about the potential harm that could result from immature individuals' making decisions about drinking. A further concern is the belief that "condoning" use of alcohol by underage drinkers may actually result in increased usage of alcohol among drinkers, or in a decision by abstainers to drink.

Although it may be more morally and ethically consistent to support abstinence-only programs, few people—including policy makers and college administrators—view abstinence-based programs like Drug Abuse Resistance Education (D.A.R.E.) or the "Just Say No" campaign as a viable solution to the problem of alcohol abuse among college students. And, unfortunately, this skepticism is well founded. Despite a decade of abstinence-only messages promulgated by D.A.R.E. and similar nationwide efforts, drinking rates among adolescent and young adult students have been relatively stable for some time (use of *other* drugs has, however, decreased) (Johnston et al., 1996). One way to begin addressing this dilemma is by weighing the potential social and individual benefits of providing drinking skills to underage students against the potential costs and risks (see Table 1.1).

Personal Barriers

As suggested above in the discussion of risk factors, few heavy-drinking college students view their alcohol use as excessive or potentially problematic. This can hinder their ability to perceive likely alcohol risks, and thus can decrease their motivation to reduce

TABLE 1.1. Risks and Benefits of Providing Drinking Skills to Underage Students

Costs/risks	Benefits
Teaching drinking skills may be condoning illegal behavior.	*Students who choose to drink can learn to do so safely.*
Some fear that underage drinkers may be more susceptible to breaking other laws. There is some evidence to suggest that youth who drink alcohol may be more likely to break laws than youth who don't drink. The relevant question is whether alcohol is the cause of this behavior, or is instead highly associated with a constellation of problematic behaviors. Research in the area of conduct disorder and sensation seeking supports the latter explanation. For individuals without a history of conduct disorder, it is unlikely that drinking illegally will promote other illegal behaviors.	Most young people who drink "copy" or imitate the drinking practices of their peers, who may know no more than they do about how to drink safely. From a harm reduction viewpoint, teaching drinking skills to young people who are already drinking is like teaching young people how to drive safely. Students find it difficult to "fit in" without conforming to the drinking habits of their peers within a party context. Learning how to refuse a drink effectively is another benefit of this approach.
Abstainers may initiate drinking at a faster rate than they might otherwise.	*Students who learn moderate-drinking skills reduce their alcohol consumption and report fewer alcohol problems.*
This is an empirical question. We are aware of no studies in this area. The more relevant concern is whether they initiate heavy, risky drinking at a faster rate than abstainers who do not receive this training.	Results from our empirically validated studies have consistently indicated that students who receive moderation skills drink less and report fewer problems, compared to control group students (Marlatt et al., in press).
Lighter drinkers may increase their rate (i.e., frequency and quantity) of drinking.	When allowed to choose for themselves, some students who drink may decide to abstain.
This is also a question for science. We are aware of no data to support this concern.	After receiving the brief intervention described in this manual, some students decided that drinking wasn't worth the risks they took or saw their friends take when they drank, and so decided to abstain.

hazardous drinking habits. Students typically provide one of several reasons for lack of concern about their heavy consumption patterns and related alcohol problems:

- Everyone drinks in college; it's an essential part of socializing.

- Weekend parties with alcohol are great ways to have fun and unwind after a grueling week of studying and examinations.

- They are in excellent physical health and have no intention of continuing their current pattern of use once they graduate from college.

- Drinking alcohol and partying are part of growing up, and a way to assert their freedom and independence.

- Alcohol use makes it possible to interact with potential dating partners.

- College is the last time to have fun before entering the real world of work and other adult responsibilities.

Conceptual Barriers

Conceptual barriers slowing the development of effective prevention for young people include differences of opinion about whether alcohol abuse is sometimes or always a precursor to alcohol dependence if untreated. These differences of opinion are broadly captured by the predominant models of addiction—the Twelve-Step and the disease model versus the biopsychosocial model. Advocates of the Twelve-Step and the disease model tend to view addictions in dichotomous terms (e.g., a person either has the disease of addiction or is disease-free); by contrast, proponents of the biopsychosocial model are more likely to view alcohol problems as existing along a continuum and to acknowledge that people can move back and forth along this continuum over time. Whereas the solution to alcohol problems from the Twelve-Step and disease model perspective is often complete abstinence to prevent further progression of the disease, advocates of the biopsychosocial model are more likely to draw from a wider range of treatment options, which often include moderation and other harm reduction approaches.

Although the dichotomous nature of the Twelve-Step and disease model perspective is of considerable use for many, such an approach to alcohol problems can serve as a sizable barrier to seeking assistance for many young adults. One problem with a dichotomous categorization is that it eliminates a "middle ground" for describing less chronic and severe drinking habits (Marlatt, Larimer, Baer, & Quigley, 1993; Fingerette, 1988; Sobell & Sobell, 1993). Problem drinkers, heavy drinkers, binge drinkers, and alcoholics are assumed to be generally alike, with a predictable downhill course unless the drinkers adopt a lifestyle of steadfast abstinence. Not surprisingly, this type of problem formulation ends up alienating many of those with less chronic conditions who may be more amenable to a brief intervention. In addition, many alcohol abusing college students find themselves "not relating" either to Alcoholics Anonymous or to the need for abstinence. Because of their lack of extensive problems or a lengthy drinking history, and because of the normative nature of heavy drinking among their same-age peers, most heavy-drinking college students see themselves as distinctly different from persons with chronic alcohol histories and related life problems. Finding little in common with these persons, alcohol-abusing young adults are likely to reject being labeled as "alcoholics" and are likely to avoid affiliation with people and organizations that make use of these labels.

MOVING PAST BARRIERS AND TOWARD A SCIENTIFICALLY INFORMED APPROACH

A report by the Institute of Medicine (1990) has argued in favor of broadening the base of treatment for alcohol problems by moving beyond treatment of chronic alcohol

• • •

dependence to prevention of alcohol abuse and early intervention for targeted at-risk groups (e.g., college students). This report has further advised that efforts be made to match particular clients to particular prevention and treatment programs, in order to increase the probability of success. **"Treatment matching"** is based on the notion that a spectrum of alcohol consumption and related problems exists (see Figure 1.1); that no single treatment approach is effective in treating all persons with alcohol problems; and that different programs may be optimal for different types of people. Individual characteristics considered in matching can include age, gender, severity of symptoms, beliefs about treatment, and other personality characteristics (Mattson & Allen, 1991).

Echoing many of the tenets of the Institute of Medicine report, Miller and Hester (1995, p. 8) recommend replacing the predominant myths about alcohol treatment ("Nothing Works," "One approach is superior to all others," and "All treatment approaches work equally well") with a practice of **informed eclecticism.** Described as "an openness to a variety of approaches that is guided by scientific evidence," the central assertions of informed eclecticism include the following:

1. There is no single superior treatment approach that works across the board for all individuals.

2. Treatment programs should make use of a multimodal approach that integrates different treatment methods shown to be effective.

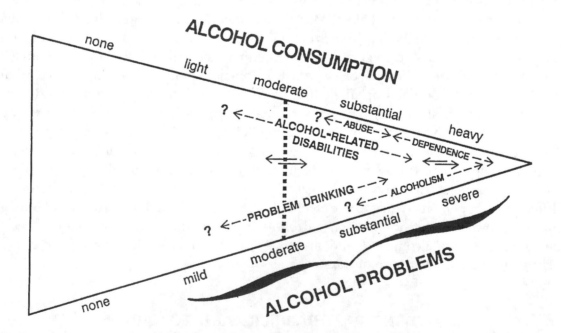

FIGURE 1.1. Spectrum of alcohol consumption and related alcohol problems. From Institute of Medicine (1990). Reprinted with permission from *Broadening the Base of Treatment for Alcohol Problems.* Copyright 1990 by the National Academy of Sciences. Courtesy of the National Academy Press, Washington, DC.

3. Different types of individuals respond best to different treatments and different kinds of approaches.

4. It is possible to match clients to treatment approaches in ways that increase the probability of treatment effectiveness and efficiency.

Consistent with these views, the indicated preventive intervention described in this manual is based on state-of-the-art empirically validated prevention and treatment approaches for alcohol problems. BASICS is tailored to the specific needs of young college student drinkers and has been developed on the basis of numerous studies (our own and other alcohol researchers') of this specific population. As clinical researchers, we acknowledge the multiple influencing factors in the etiology of alcohol problems, as well as the weight and seriousness of the barriers to prevention and treatment described above. Thus, BASICS focuses on empirically derived personal risk factors and other individual characteristics relevant to treatment. We seek to stay clear of discussions and philosophical debates about the "causes" of addictions within the context of the intervention, and instead focus on pragmatic strategies and approaches that have been shown to reduce alcohol consumption and related negative consequences among a population of students already drinking alcohol in considerably risky ways. More specifically, because the majority of heavy-drinking college students are expected to "mature out" of problematic patterns of consumption as they move through their 20s, our aim is to accelerate the rate of this maturation through efforts to enhance students' motivation to reduce drinking risks and through skill building.

Following the Institute of Medicine's (1990) recommendations, we meet each student on his or her own terms by using a brief motivational intervention to encourage moderate, less risky use of alcohol if the student chooses to drink. Students who are severely alcohol-dependent, who have been advised by a physician not to drink, or who have medical conditions in which use of alcohol may be contraindicated (e.g., possible pregnancy, ulcers, diabetes, etc.) are encouraged to abstain from alcohol use, to seek a medical consultation, and/or to accept referral to an abstinence-based program.

CHAPTER 2

The Alcohol Skills Training Program

C ognitive-behavioral programs for alcohol abusers have generated encouraging results—in particular, reductions in various alcohol-related consequences (see Hester & Miller, 1995, for a review of effective cognitive and behavioral approaches to alcohol problems; see also Alden, 1988, and Sanchez-Craig, Annis, Bornet, & MacDonald, 1984). College students who are heavy drinkers need specific skills and practice in order to change their high-risk drinking behavior. For example, although students might recognize that their pattern of heavy drinking poses certain dangers or risks, they may be unable or unwilling to reduce their consumption unless they feel they can develop alternative coping strategies to counteract the social pressures and other factors that motivate them to drink.

For over a decade, the Addictive Behaviors Research Center at the University of Washington has developed and empirically tested various alcohol prevention programs for high-risk college drinkers. These programs are based on cognitive-behavioral skills training and motivational enhancement strategies (Baer, Kivlahan, Fromme, & Marlatt, 1989; Marlatt et al., 1998; Kivlahan, Marlatt, Fromme, Coppel, & Williams, 1990; Baer, 1993; Dimeff, 1997). Although the modalities themselves are quite distinct, together they constitute a core curriculum that we have named the Alcohol Skills Training Program (ASTP). The main conceptual components of ASTP, the specific ASTP modalities, and results from controlled outcome research studies are described below.

CONCEPTUAL BACKGROUND OF THE PROGRAM

ASTP was developed largely in response to the limited success of other prevention programs during the mid-1980s in changing students' drinking behavior and reducing alcohol-related risks. The key elements underlying the ASTP approach include (1) the application of cognitive-behavioral self-management strategies (based on the relapse prevention model), (2) the use of motivational enhancement techniques, and (3) the use of harm reduction principles.

Although relapse prevention was initially developed as a maintenance program for the treatment of addictive behaviors (Marlatt & Gordon, 1980, 1985), the cognitive and behavioral strategies of relapse prevention have been extended to facilitate many positive lifestyle changes that reduce health risks, including physical disease, psychological distress, and the development of addictive behaviors (Dimeff & Marlatt, 1995; Marlatt & George, 1984). In the context of ASTP, these strategies aim to change drinking behavior and associated lifestyle habits through enhancing the effectiveness of coping responses, building and bolstering skills, and increasing self-efficacy for behavioral self-management. Except in the case of severe alcohol dependence, goals are tailored to the needs of the individual. Students are encouraged to build a balanced lifestyle. "Healthy addictions," such as aerobic exercise, meditation, and other stress-reducing practices, are encouraged.

Like that of other skills-based training programs, the content of ASTP is based primarily on cognitive-behavioral strategies, such as setting drinking limits, monitoring one's drinking, rehearsing drink refusal, and practicing other useful new behaviors through role play. Traditionally, skills training programs are built on the assumption that the client enters therapy with the intended purpose of changing a particular behavior or set of behaviors. Motivation to change the behavior is assumed. Consider, for example, a socially awkward and shy young man who seeks therapy to decrease his debilitating social anxiety and increase his dating negotiation skills, or a woman with a 20-year history of cigarette smoking who seeks skills to help manage urges and cravings to smoke as she embarks on giving up her habit. In both these scenarios, the individuals are fully aware of the need to find more effective ways of acting and responding. Furthermore, both are eager to make behavioral changes at the outset of treatment.

Unlike the individuals in these scenarios, college students who drink hazardously or who have experienced problems because of their alcohol use seldom identify their behavior as risky or problematic. Rarely do these students seek treatment or other assistance of their own accord. For this reason, we have departed slightly from traditional skills training programs by embedding our skills training in a context of motivation building. We employ motivational interviewing strategies, which were originally developed by William R. Miller at the University of New Mexico, in an effort to create and bolster "readiness and eagerness" to change (Miller & Rollnick, 1991).

The role of motivation in effecting change in young adults' drinking patterns must be considered in any efforts at prevention programming for this population. College students are usually well informed about the risks of alcohol and drug use through repeated exposure to various prevention efforts, from high school health classes to "Just Say No" television commercials. In addition, most students are quite capable of "saying no" if they desire to do so. As a result, information and skills are useful only to the extent that the students make use of the skills. To illustrate this point, many college drinkers are well aware of the hazards of drinking and driving. Many have grown up hearing warnings about drunk driving through the successful grassroots campaign efforts of Mothers Against Drunk Driving, Students Against Drunk Driving, and other organizations; they can probably recall previously learned behavioral strategies to avoid these risks (e.g., designating a sober driver prior to the drinking occasion, turning car keys over to a nondrinking friend or designated driver, calling a taxi, etc.). Despite their awareness of these hazards and prevention strategies, many still drive shortly after drinking, or willingly ride with someone they know is intoxicated. From a motivational perspective, the goal is to increase the students' interest in making the necessary lifestyle changes that increase the probability that they will put the skills to use.

As previously noted, ASTP is also based on harm reduction principles. This approach has been widely used in AIDS education programs to promote the use of condoms and safer sex practices, and in needle exchange programs, where injection drug users receive clean needles, syringes, and bleach for cleaning needles; all of these efforts are intended to reduce new cases of HIV infection (Marlatt, 1998a; Erickson, Riley, Cheung, & O'Hare, 1997; Marlatt & Tapert, 1993). Harm reduction methods are based on the assumption that addictive behaviors, including alcohol abuse and alcohol dependence, can be placed along a continuum of harmful consequences. The primary goal of harm reduction is to facilitate movement along this continuum from more to less harmful effects. Although abstinence is considered the anchor point of minimal harm, any incremental movement toward reduced harm is encouraged and supported.

Diane Riley (1994), of the Canadian Centre on Substance Abuse, has defined harm reduction this way:

> The first priority of harm reduction is to decrease the negative consequences of drug use. By contrast, drug policy in North America has traditionally focused on reducing the prevalence of drug use. Harm reduction establishes a hierarchy of goals, with the most immediate and realistic ones to be achieved as first steps toward risk-free use, or if appropriate, abstinence.
>
> Drug-taking behaviors result in effects that are either beneficial (as in the case of life-saving medication), neutral, or harmful. Assigning a positive or negative value—a benefit or harm—to such effects is subjective and open to controversy, but a harm reduction framework at least offers a pragmatic means by which consequences can be objectively evaluated. (p. 1)

Controlled drinking in the treatment of alcohol abuse and dependence is one example of the application of harm reduction within the alcohol field (see Marlatt et al., 1993, for a review of the controlled-drinking research literature and related controversy). Briefly, controlled drinking, or moderation training, provides an effective alternative to abstinence for alcohol-abusing or mildly alcohol-dependent individuals who are interested in changing their pattern of drinking, but choose not to abstain. Specific, nonabusive drinking guidelines are established as the treatment goal. With the exception of different treatment goals, cognitive-behavioral treatment progresses in a fashion similar to that for those choosing abstinence: identifying factors that correspond to violations of the treatment goal, and developing compensatory skills to manage these high-risk situations more effectively.

ASTP MODALITIES

We have generated and empirically evaluated three separate indicated prevention modalities based on ASTP: (1) a student correspondence course manual; (2) a multi-session Alcohol Skills Training Course; and (3) BASICS. These programs are designed to be used either separately or in combination with other prevention strategies.

Student Correspondence Course Manual

The first modality consists of a self-guided instructional manual, *The Alcohol Skills Training Manual* (Baer, Kivlahan, et al., 1991) containing six units. Each unit of this manual includes graphs and diagrams of important points, "new ideas," and exercises that elaborate important unit points (e.g., determining one's positive alcohol expectancies, practicing refusing drinks, and experimenting with having fun at a party while not drinking). The obvious advantage of this program is that it is self-contained and does not require instruction. The obvious disadvantage is that it requires considerable initiative and motivation to complete.

Alcohol Skills Training Course

The second modality is a six- to eight-session course taught by a trained instructor. The course uses brief didactic presentations and small-group discussions; the student manual described above can be used as a text adjunct to the group experience. Exercises consist of class dialogues and demonstrations, including role playing. The course includes a discussion of models of addiction and a placebo drinking experience in a simulated bar, followed by a discussion of the role of expectancies in alcohol consumption. The classroom format provides a number of advantages. For one thing, positive peer relations develop as the group collectively challenges the "party" norms of other peers and develops alternatives to these norms. Peer influence is maximized to achieve this end. In addition, young adult men and women learn what others truly find attractive in a partner as a way to debunk alcohol myths. As is the case in most interactive groups, participants also learn from the knowledge and applied experience of their peers. As a result of all these factors, participants develop a broader range of information and skills than they might do in one-on-one sessions that focus specifically on what proves "relevant" to them and their lifestyles at the time of the preventive intervention. *The Alcohol Skills Training Manual* used in the correspondence cause serves as the workbook for this modality.

Brief Alcohol Screening and Intervention for College Students

Of the three skills training approaches that constitute ASTP, BASICS is the briefest and potentially most cost-effective method. Based on the Brief Drinker's Check-Up (Miller & Sovereign, 1989), BASICS consists of two 50-minute sessions (with an additional 50 minutes after or before the first session for the completion of self-report measures). The purpose of the first session is to assess an individual student's drinking pattern, related attitudes about alcohol, and motivation to change drinking; the purpose of the second session is to provide the student with feedback about his or her personal risk factors and advice about ways to moderate drinking. The student also receives computer-generated personalized graphic feedback summarizing the reviewed material. Although it is considerably briefer than the other two modalities, BASICS nonetheless combines information about alcohol effects, identification of personal risk factors, discussion of specific cognitive and behavioral strategies to moderate drinking, and motivational enhancement strategies aimed at building interest in changing heavy-drinking behavior (Miller & Rollnick, 1990).

As is true of the other ASTP modalities, information about alcohol and related risks is embedded within a broader frame of lifestyle behaviors in the brief intervention. There are a number of compelling reasons to examine alcohol consumption within this broader context:

1. Students are far more receptive to information and feedback about alcohol when the topic of alcohol is part of a larger discussion of lifestyle or health habits.

2. There is reason to believe that a broader range of health behaviors may be needed to predict and prevent alcohol abuse in young adult women, given the correlation of heavy drinking with disordered eating and psychological distress in college women (Perkins, 1992).

3. Because it incorporates other lifestyle behaviors, this preventive intervention can "fit" more compatibly within a wellness program approach, now popular at many colleges.

More than the other two ASTP modalities, BASICS draws upon the literature on brief interventions, which have a rich data base demonstrating their effectiveness in treating alcohol problems. The history of brief interventions began with early studies by Orford, Oppenheimer, and Edwards (1976), who found that brief contact with a respected medical professional (in this case, a physician) was as effective as 2 weeks of inpatient hospitalization for alcoholism, particularly for those with less severe dependence. Subsequent studies have typically found brief interventions to be more effective than no treatment at all, frequently as effective as more extensive treatments, and likely to enhance the effectiveness of subsequent treatment (see Bien, Miller, & Tonigan, 1993, and Heather, 1995, for reviews). A recent methodological analysis of alcohol treatment outcome studies conducted by Miller, Brown, et al. (1995) found that brief interventions had "one of the largest literature bases and currently the most positive" (p. 22).

A **brief intervention** is typically defined as minimal interaction with a medical or mental health professional focusing on the health risks associated with drinking, and ranging from several minutes in length up to several sessions. Brief interventions are particularly effective for individuals like most heavy-drinking college students, who do not have severe alcohol dependence, but who are nonetheless having minimal to moderate alcohol problems or who drink in harmful, hazardous ways (Institute of Medicine, 1990). Because brief interventions are as effective as more intensive treatments for individuals who are not severely alcohol-dependent, such interventions can be realistic (e.g., cost-effective) ways of providing services to more individuals, while saving resources for more intensive treatments (e.g., intensive outpatient and inpatient) for those requiring such treatments.

Miller and Rollnick (1991) use the acronym "FRAMES" to capture the active ingredients of brief interventions with demonstrated effectiveness:

- **Feedback**—information about current health status, risks, normative behavior.

- **Responsibility**—emphasis placed on the client's responsibility for change.

- **Advice**—simple advice on what to change (e.g., hazardous drinking), suggestions for moderation.

- **Menu** (of treatment options)—provision of a range of options to select from.

- **Empathy**—ability to see the situation from the client's perspective, while also maintaining a foot outside his or her reality.

- **Self-efficacy**—the client's belief in his or her ability to make successful changes.

Brief interventions have most commonly been employed within the context of primary care and provided by nurses and physicians. Numerous studies have found physician-based interventions to be effective, low-cost approaches for bringing about changes in a variety of health behaviors: cessation or moderation of heavy drinking (World Health Organization [WHO] Brief Intervention Study Group, 1996; Fleming, Barry, Manwell, Johnson, & London, 1997; Babor, 1990; Allen, Maisto, & Connors, 1995; Bradley, 1992; Wallace, Cutler, & Haines, 1988; Anderson & Scott, 1992; Strecher, Kobrin, Kreuter, Roodhouse, & Farrell, 1994); smoking cessation (Strecher et al., 1994; Manley, Epps, & Glynn, 1992; Gilpin, Pierce, Johnson, & Bal, 1993; Ockene, 1987; Cohen, Stookey, Katz, Brook, & Smith, 1989); improvement in dietary behavior (Campbell et al., 1994; Curry, Kristal, & Bowen, 1992); and more diligent cancer prevention efforts (Skinner, Strecher, & Hospers, 1994; McPhee, Bird, Fordham, Rodnick, & Osborn, 1991).

The most comprehensive primary care brief intervention study to date, the WHO Collaborative Project on Identification and Treatment of Persons with Harmful Alcohol

Consumption, recently released results from its eight-nation study with heavy drinkers (WHO Brief Intervention Study Group, 1996). This study compared two brief interventions against an assessment-only control group to test the minimum and the maximum amount of effort primary care workers could be expected to devote per patient visit to the topic of heavy drinking. Over 1,500 patients were randomly assigned to either an assessment-only condition, simple advice, or brief counseling. Both interventions were administered by professionals within the primary care setting, including nurses (46.3%) and physicians (17.3%). Patients in both intervention conditions received a problem-solving manual describing the benefits of moderate drinking or abstinence, ways of coping with high-risk drinking situations, and constructive alternatives to drinking. In addition, simple advice included a brief discussion of sensible drinking limits, whereas patients receiving the other brief intervention were provided with 15 minutes of counseling about their use of alcohol. Although it was hypothesized that reductions in alcohol consumption would be proportional to the intervention's intensity, no differences were observed between the two brief intervention groups at the 9-month follow-up. Both interventions proved effective for men in reducing the average rate of consumption and intensity of drinking, in comparison to the control condition. Although significant reductions in drinking were observed for women in all three conditions, no differences between groups were observed.

In light of the consistent success of brief interventions, the Institute of Medicine (1990) has recommended use of a stepped-care approach to treatment, in which minimal efforts are provided initially and the intensity of treatment is increased only if the minimal efforts prove unsuccessful. Originally used as an approach to medical treatment for hypertension (Sobell & Sobell, 1993), stepped care requires that the least invasive course of treatment commensurate with the problem's severity be initiated first. If the therapeutic effect is not achieved, treatment is then titrated up. For example, a patient diagnosed with borderline diabetes is initially prescribed a diet to stabilize his or her blood sugar level before insulin injections are considered. Similarly, a college student presenting with symptoms of alcohol abuse receives a brief intervention before more extensive treatment measures are taken, such as admitting the client to an alcohol rehabilitation program. Should the client have difficulty achieving the desired treatment outcome, he or she may then be "bumped up" a notch to weekly group therapy for alcohol abusers. This approach naturally requires that the practitioner have a menu of stepped-care options and referrals to select from, should a client desire or need additional assistance.

Brief interventions often make use of personalized graphic summaries that illustrate an individual's health risks, based on previously gathered self-report data. Providing people with their test results or other technical information in written form can contribute to increased comprehension and retention of the material. This personalized feedback can also provide a structure or outline for discussions with clients about their behavior. Commonly used in brief interventions, personalized graphic feedback often includes a summary of drinking habits, a comparison of drinking habits to general norms, risk factors (e.g., family history, degree of alcohol dependence), results of medical or psychological assessment (e.g., liver function, neuropsychological or cognitive impairment from heavy drinking), and cognitive factors (e.g., beliefs about the common effects from drinking).

Agostinelli and her colleagues at the University of New Mexico (Agostinelli, Brown, & Miller, 1995) recently conducted a pilot study of a brief motivational feedback intervention for heavy-drinking college students, which relied solely on mailing participants personalized graphic feedback prepared on the basis of a mail-in paper-and-pencil assessment. Students who volunteered to participate in this study were randomly assigned to either the brief intervention group or an assessment-only control condition. Students receiving the brief intervention were mailed personalized graphic feedback similar in content to the feedback provided in BASICS. Feedback included percentile ranking comparing a student's typical pattern of alcohol use in the preceding 60 days to U.S. population norms; estimated peak blood alcohol level (BAL); and a summary of personal risk factors, including tolerance to alcohol and family history. Although lacking in stringent internal validity controls, this study demonstrated that students receiving this minimal mail-in intervention showed greater reductions in weekly consumption and in typical intoxication levels than controls did. Results from this study suggest that an intervention far more minimal than BASICS can achieve significant reductions in drinking rates among high-risk college drinkers.

Personalized feedback can be built into a computerized assessment as the individual proceeds or a printed feedback form can be generated after the completion of the assessment (see Chapter 5 and Appendix B of the present manual). Such feedback is standard practice within motivational enhancement therapy (Miller, Zweben, DiClemente, & Rychtarik, 1992; Miller & Rollnick, 1991). Care providers can make use of the printed feedback as a medical doctor makes use of laboratory test results when reviewing these findings with a patient.

OVERVIEW OF RESEARCH FINDINGS ON ASTP

Thus far, three studies have been conducted as empirical tests of the effectiveness of ASTP. The initial study (Kivlahan et al., 1990) compared the efficacy of ASTP's eight-session Alcohol Skills Training Course for high-risk drinkers to an Alcohol Information School format modeled after the Washington State program for first-time offenders convicted of driving while intoxicated. An assessment-only control group was also included. The content of the Alcohol Information School was purely informational; no new coping skills were taught or practiced. Lecture topics included physical and behavioral effects of alcohol, dispelling myths about alcohol, alcoholism problems, and legal aspects of alcoholism. Students assigned to the control condition participated in all baseline and follow-up assessment procedures, but received no prevention program until after the completion of the 1-year follow-up period. At baseline, students reported an average of 15 drinks per week and an estimated peak weekly BAL of 0.13% (0.10% or above defines legal intoxication for driving in most states). At the 1-year follow-up, ASTP subjects reported 6.6 drinks weekly and a peak BAL of 0.07%, compared to 12.7 drinks per week and a peak BAL of 0.09% for students in the Alcohol Information School condition, and 16.8 drinks per week and a 0.11% peak blood-alcohol level for the control condition. Other drinking measures showed that students receiving the ASTP had reduced their drinking significantly more than subjects in the other two conditions at the 1-year follow-up.

The second study (Baer et al., 1989, 1992) replicated the first study and compared the effectiveness of the three ASTP modalities: the Alcohol Skills Training Course, a 1-hour version of the BASICS brief intervention, and the manual-driven correspondence course. Students reported drinking an average of 20 drinks per week at baseline, spread across four drinking occasions. Estimated peak BAL was 0.14%, and students reported experiencing numerous problems because of drinking. As in the first study, students on average significantly reduced their alcohol consumption during the course of the study. Gains were maintained throughout 1- and 2-year follow-up periods. Average drinks per week declined overall from 12.5 to 8.5 drinks per week. Average peak BAL was also reduced from 0.14% to 0.10%. Although these findings support the efficacy of all three modalities, we are particularly enthusiastic about the outcome effects of the BASICS feedback component, for several important reasons: This condition appears to be the most likely to be completed, potentially the most cost-effective, and the most easily tailored to an individual's risks and degree of readiness for commencing with a program of behavior change.

The Lifestyles Project (Baer, 1993; Marlatt et al., 1998) was designed to replicate and extend our earlier studies of brief harm reduction programs with heavy-drinking college students. Briefly, 2,157 incoming freshmen were screened as seniors in high school for purposes of participation in a 4-year longitudinal study. The 508 students deemed most at risk for alcohol problems were selected to participate in the study. Risk criteria included a pattern of heavy alcohol consumption at the time of the initial screening or a history of problems resulting from alcohol use. Of these 508, 366 were ultimately recruited and were randomly assigned to either an experimental or a high-risk control condition. An additional 150 students were selected from the larger pool as a control group that would enable us to observe the natural course of drinking patterns among college students. Subjects assigned to the experimental condition received BASICS in addition to the assessment procedure. All other subjects received the assessment procedure only.

Although high-risk drinkers in both the experimental and control conditions reported a mean decrease in consumption of alcohol at the 1- and 2-year follow-ups, students receiving BASICS made significantly greater reductions in their use. Furthermore, students receiving BASICS reported significantly fewer alcohol-related problems as measured by the Rutgers Alcohol Problems Inventory (White & Labouvie, 1989), and fewer symptoms of alcohol dependence as measured by the Alcohol Dependence Scale (Skinner & Horn, 1984), compared to students in the high-risk control condition. Although statistically significant decrements were found for both alcohol consumption and drinking problems, the magnitude of the treatment effect was greater for drinking problems. This suggests that amount consumed and alcohol-related problems may be correlated, but they may not be causally related. This finding is of considerable importance, to the extent that it suggests that indicated prevention programs may be least effective if they only focus on reducing or eliminating drinking as opposed to addressing proximal harmful effects. Treatment × time interactions are summarized in Figure 2.1 for drinking rates and problems.

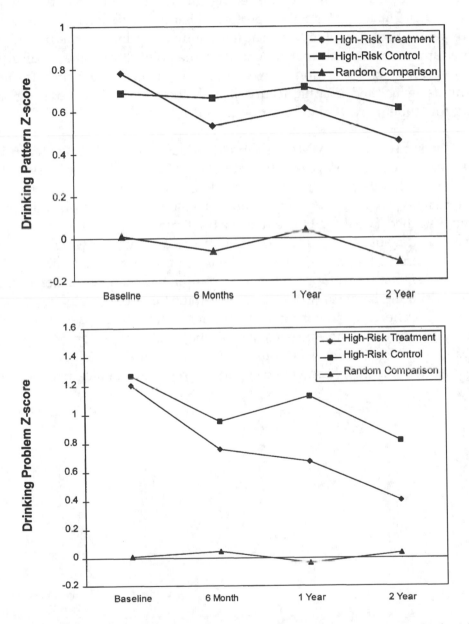

FIGURE 2.1. Z-transformed problem rates over time for high-risk treatment, high-risk control, and random comparison groups. From Marlatt (1998a). Copyright 1998 by the American Psychological Association. Reprinted by permission.

We sought to develop and assess the feasibility of a streamlined version of Marlatt's BASICS for use in a student health center and to test its efficacy (Dimeff & McNeely, in press; Dimeff, 1997). Our interest in this project was precipitated by recognition that most colleges and universities would be financially unable to implement the full BASICS intervention with more than a handful of students given the prevalence of heavy and hazardous drinking among college students. Additionally, student health centers typically serve a large proportion of the student population during the course of the academic year. To achieve the goal of streamlining BASICS to meet the pragmatic needs and resources of a primary care setting, we developed the Multi-Media Assessment of Student Health (MMASH) to perform the initial assessment and automatically generate personalized graphic feedback for use by the primary care provider during his or her appointment with the student. At some point during the medical appointment, the primary care practitioner would spend between 3 to 5 minutes reviewing the computer-generated graphic feedback with the student and advising moderate drinking for students who plan to continue to drink.

In the pilot study trial of MMASH, undergraduate students seeking services at a student health center were asked to complete MMASH (Dimeff, 1997). Students meeting high risk criteria for heavy or hazardous drinking were invited to participate in the research program. Forty-one students volunteered to participate and were randomly assigned by MMASH to either the brief intervention experimental condition or a treatment-as-usual control condition. Immediately following completion of MMASH, experimental participants and their primary care practitioner received and reviewed a personalized graphic feedback from an attached computer that summarized their drinking habits and risks, and encouraged moderate drinking. Moderate to large treatment effect sizes favoring the brief intervention were observed on self-report measures of binge drinking episodes and alcohol problems at the 30-day follow-up. Statistically significant gains were observed among those participants receiving the most exposure to the intervention in comparison to those who receiving less exposure.

CHAPTER 3

Laying the Foundations for BASICS

*I*n the first part of this chapter, we aim to familiarize the reader with relevant clinical approaches to addictive behaviors used in BASICS. Specifically, we examine the central components of motivational interviewing (particularly the stages-of-change model for understanding the process of behavior change) and of cognitive-behavioral skills training. In addition to providing a review, we explore the similarities and differences of these approaches, and describe how we have applied them to BASICS. Following this review, we next discuss the basic information about alcohol that is provided to clients in BASICS. We conclude the chapter with a brief review of the specific clinical aims of BASICS, issues relevant to therapist–treatment matching and student recruitment, and the BASICS format.

Theoretical Approaches to Preventing Harm from Alcohol Use

What's in a Model?
Models of Helping and Coping
Motivational Interviewing
Cognitive-Behavioral Approach to High-Risk Behaviors
Integrating Motivational Interviewing and Cognitive-Behavioral Skills Training

Basic Information about Alcohol

Positive Alcohol Expectancies
Debunking the Myth that "More Is Better": The Biphasic Effect
Alcohol Myopia
Differential Risks for Women and Men
Blood Alcohol Effects
Tolerance
The Detrimental Effects of Alcohol Intoxication on Sleep, Alertness, and Performance

BASICS Clinical Aims, Therapist/Client Issues, and Format

Aims of BASICS
Clinical Approach in BASICS

• • •

Therapist Matching to BASICS
How Students Are Recruited
The BASICS Format
The Primary Components of Sessions 1 and 2

THEORETICAL APPROACHES TO PREVENTING HARM FROM ALCOHOL USE

The theoretical underpinning for BASICS is reviewed in this section. We begin with a brief discussion of why it is functionally necessary for clinicians to consider their beliefs about the causes of addictions. We then review the predominant models of addictions in the United States today and examine some of the assumptions on which they are built. Next, we provide a brief overview of motivational interviewing, a brief intervention approach aimed at moving people through the stages-of-change continuum (a concept developed by James Prochaska and Carlo DiClemente, and also discussed here). Finally, because BASICS takes a cognitive-behavioral skills training approach to the prevention of alcohol problems in college students, this approach and its links to Marlatt and Gordon's relapse prevention are reviewed.

What's in a Model?

Clinicians' beliefs about high-risk or addictive behaviors usually bear heavily on how treatment is approached and how clients' behaviors are understood. Although a number of models for understanding these behaviors have existed for some time, the field has been divided between academics with one model in mind and treatment providers working "in the trenches" with a different model in mind. These differences in opinion about the causes of addictions were viewed by many as directly threatening the field as a whole. This division of allegiances made it difficult to share information and wisdom in an effort to develop effective treatments for a diversity of clients with numerous and varied problems. Because models, like theories, are conceptual attempts to explain reality, they contain assumptions about how things work. Sometimes the assumptions are supported by the data, and other times they are not. Problems tend to arise when clinicians are in a sense blind to the assumptions they are making and fail to recognize that some assumptions are not supported by the clinical data. For this reason, we encourage therapists to consider their assumptions about addictive behaviors and about how people make changes. As it turns out, this is particularly important when working with young people, whose reasons for drinking and whose drinking styles are very different from those of older adults.

Models of Helping and Coping

In their two-factor attributional analysis of helping and coping, Brickman (1983) examined four principal models based on determinants of etiology and determinants of behavior change. When applied to addictive behaviors, each model is an attempt to answer two central questions: (1) Is the addict/alcoholic responsible for the development of the problem (etiology), and (2) is the addict/alcoholic responsible for changing the problem? When placed in a 2 × 2 matrix, the four models provide a general framework for understanding addiction problems and a jumping-off point for considering approaches to prevention, treatment, and relapse (Dimeff & Marlatt, 1995; Marlatt & Gordon, 1985). The four models are as follows: the moral model, the disease model, the spiritual (Twelve-Step) model, and the biopsychosocial habit model (see Figure 3.1).

The moral model assumes that the individual is responsible for the development of the addiction problem, as well as for changing or failing to change the addictive behavior. Failure to change or relapse is believed to be caused by a lack of willpower. Implicit in this model is the belief that addicted persons have the capacity to overcome their plight if only they are interested in doing so or possess sufficient moral fiber. Unfortunately, this perspective often results in a "blaming the victim" mentality.

In contrast, the disease model posits that an addiction is a manifestation of an underlying disease process rooted in an individual's genetic or physiological makeup. The addict is often told that there is no cure for the disease and that the affliction is progressive in nature; unless total abstinence is achieved, the person will follow a downward path toward despair, death, or "the gates of insanity." Like the diabetic who must resist the craving to eat sugar lest he or she experience a seizure or death, the addict must resist all use of the addictive substance. In its purest form, the disease

Responsible for Changing Problem?

(Is person capable of changing without self-help or treament group?)

		YES	NO
YES Personally Responsible for Developing an Addictive Behavior? **NO**		Moral Model *(Relapse = Sin)*	Spiritual (Twelve-Step) Model *(Relapse = Loss of Contact with Higher Power)*
		Biopsychosocial Habit Model *(Relapse = Mistake/Error)*	Disease Model *(Relapse = Reactivation of Progressive Disease)*

FIGURE 3.1. Models of addiction and relapse: Brickman and colleagues' attributional analysis. Adapted from Marlatt and Gordon (1985). Copyright 1985 by The Guilford Press. Adapted by permission.

model is conceptualized in these medical terms. The disease model is also used to describe a constitutional or predispositional makeup that is not necessarily biological in origin, but that results in a clear demarcation between addicts/alcoholics and "normals." Specific assumptions of the disease model that differentiate it from the biopsychosocial model include the following (Mercer & Woody, 1992):

1. Addiction is a chronic and progressive disease that has predictable symptoms and a predictable course, starting with abuse of the substance.

2. Addicts and alcoholics have permanently lost the capacity to control their use of substances and alcohol.

3. Addiction affects an addict's body, mind, and spirit; as such, recovery from addictions involves a lifelong process of healing in each of these areas.

4. Because of the nature of the disease, the only viable option for addicts is total, lifelong abstinence.

5. Addicts and alcoholics will have the best chance of maintaining sobriety and abstinence by accepting that they have a disease that produces a loss of control over drugs and alcohol, and if they reach out to other addicts and alcoholics through Twelve-Step programs (see below).

In many ways, the disease model addresses some of the shortcomings of the moral model by freeing the addicted individual from blame for having an addiction. Unfortunately, a price is paid for this tradeoff. Because of the claim that a disease process is at fault and/or that the individual is constitutionally constructed to have an addiction problems, the person can never look forward to a time when he or she is "recovered." Instead, the addict must forever fears the resurgence or activation of the disease state. Just as a diabetic patient does have some personal control over managing the disease state, the addicted client can heed the warnings or other recovering addicts and alcoholics of professionals to abstain. However, again like the diabetic patient, the addict is actually believed to have only limited control over regulating the disease. In other words, something or someone other than the patient is viewed as holding power over the disease and its cure. Obviously, the drawback of this approach is that it decreases the addict's ultimate sense of personal mastery or self-efficacy in addressing the problem.

The spiritual (Twelve-Step) model considers the addict as somewhat personally responsible for his or her addiction, as a result of alienation from spiritual pursuits or engagement in sinful behaviors (which include excessive use of alcohol or other use of addictive drugs). Although the person is viewed as responsible for the fall from grace, the ultimate solution to his or her problems can only come through a spiritual source (e.g., a Higher Power, God, a Twelve-Step group, etc.). As in the disease model, the patient is needed to "show up," but the actual forces responsible for the spiritual cure are understood as outside the patient's ultimate control. In Twelve-Step programs such as Alcoholics Anonymous and Narcotics Anonymous, the addict is viewed as a self-centered individual who has often placed his or her own needs first before the needs of others or the community. The addict takes steps toward recovery by making amends to those harmed by selfish aims and greed, and by turning his or her life (including personal control over alcohol or drugs) over to a Higher Power. From this perspective, a relapse is understood as an alienation from the Higher Power.

The biopsychosocial habit model rests on the assumption that the problems experienced by an individual are not substantially of his or her own making. These problems are instead assumed to be multiply determined; they may include biological, psychological, and social factors as primary contributors to alcoholism or addiction. Although the individual is not seen as personally responsible for the cause of the problems, he or she is believed to be fully capable, with assistance, of making changes in behavior. In this way, this model recognizes the client's power and influence in the process of change. BASICS favors this model both because it allows for a multidetermined understanding of etiology and risk, and because it emphasizes the client's ability to learn more effective coping strategies to address life's challenges, including addictive behaviors.

Motivational Interviewing

Motivational interviewing is premised on the idea that motivation is dynamic and ever-changing, and not a personality trait that a person either has or lacks, or a pattern of behavior that a person is likely to move into and out of. Consider the common practice of making New Year's resolutions. The fact that many of us wait until this particular momentous occasion—the changing of the year—to undertake a particular change reflects the ambivalence that we commonly feel around this time. Despite good intentions and an energetic start, our motivation often wanes as time progresses. Unless something should "boost" or "ignite" our motivation again, it is unlikely that our target goals will be reached any time soon. When motivation is viewed as a state, the practitioner's role is clear: to assist in reigniting the original motivational spark, to provide the boost that will encourage continued effort toward the goal, and to help a client keep his or her motivation to change in top shape.

Motivational interviewing was developed specifically to facilitate change along a continuum and to help people work through their ambivalence about changing addictive or high-risk behavior (see Miller & Rollnick, 1991, for a full discussion of motivational interviewing). Describing the central aims of motivational interviewing, Rollnick, Heather, and Bell (1992) note:

> It is based upon the assumption that most patients do not enter the consultation in a state of readiness to change their patterns of drinking, smoking, exercise, diet or drug use;

therefore, straightforward advice-giving will be of limited value and will lead to the kind of non-constructive dialogue often encountered in the addictions field: the interviewer's arguments for change are met by resistance from the patient. In contrast, this method aims to help patients articulate for themselves the reasons for concern and the arguments for change. Even if a decision to change is not made in the consultation, this time will be well spent since behavior change itself could well occur in the near future. (p. 25)

Motivational interviewing matches an intervention to a client's readiness for change, because introducing action-based interventions "prematurely" (i.e., before the client is ready to change) may produce psychological reactance (Brehm & Brehm, 1981). Such reactance increases the client's defensiveness and psychological resistance to change, and thus decreases the overall effectiveness of the intervention as the client seeks to maintain psychological autonomy or personal freedom. The practitioner is instead encouraged to explore the conflict with ambivalent clients, and to encourage these clients to express their own reasons for concern and provide their own reasons for change (Rollnick, Heather, & Bell, 1992).

The overarching task of the practitioner in motivational interviewing is to actively develop and bolster a client's interest and motivation to change his or her behavior in a particular direction. Miller and Rollnick (1991) utilize Prochaska and DiClemente's stages-of-change model (Prochaska, DiClemente, & Norcross, 1992; Prochaska & DiClemente, 1984, 1986) to conceptualize this movement. Five stages are described in this model: precontemplation, contemplation, preparation, action, and maintenance.

Precontemplation is the stage in which the person is unaware (or underaware) of risks or problems associated with a particular behavior—in the present case, hazardous drinking. Persons in this stage have no intention to change their behavior in the foreseeable future. High risk college drinkers are often in this stage. In our experience, students who are required to receive an alcohol evaluation or brief intervention as a result of disciplinary action are usually in the precontemplation stage. While acknowledging that they drink heavily in comparison to other college student drinkers they know, they do not view their drinking as something in need of change. The fact that they are being required to seek professional evaluation is often interpreted by them as "bad luck" or misfortune, not as an indicator of hazardous or problematic alcohol use.

Contemplation is the stage in which the person begins to recognize that some hazards and/or problems exist and gives thought to making a change in his or her behavior, but has not yet made a firm commitment to change. This stage is primarily characterized by ambivalence about changing. While recognizing some maladaptive aspects of alcohol use, the person wavers back and forth between interest in making behavioral changes and a desire to stay put. Classic responses from students in this stage include the following:

"It's probably not so great that I keep missing my chemistry class in the morning because I'm always hung over on Thursday mornings, and, yeah, it's screwing up my GPA. However, I'm certainly not the only one who's doing this!"

"I don't think I have a problem; I'm not an alcoholic! It's just something that college students do to have fun. Maybe I should change, but I'm not sure I'm concerned enough to want to do anything about it right now."

People frequently struggle with their positive experiences while using alcohol, as well as the amount of effort, energy, and loss it will take to overcome the problem (Prochaska et al., 1992).

Preparation combines intention with behavior and usually follows once ambivalence is resolved or diminished. People in this stage have typically taken some actions in the direction of change (e.g., reduction in number of drinks consumed), but usually without a specific goal or criterion for effective action (e.g., abstaining from intoxication or abuse of alcohol). Importantly, people in the preparation stage are intent on taking deliberate action in the near future to change their behavior. Common statements heard during this stage include "I'm ready to try something else to change what I'm doing," or "I didn't realize things had gotten this far out of hand. What do you suggest?"

Action is the stage in which the client modifies his or her behavior and/or environment in order to overcome the problem. By definition, clients who have successfully altered their addictive behavior for 1 day to 6 months are classified in the action stage. Prochaska et al. (1992) caution clinicians against a myopic overemphasis on the action stage, without recognizing the process people go through to reach and sustain a behavioral goal:

> Modifications of addictive behavior made in the action stage tend to be most visible and receive the greatest external recognition. People, including professionals, often erroneously equate action with change. As a consequence, they overlook the requisite work that prepares changers for action and the important efforts necessary to maintain the changes following action. (p. 1104)

Maintenance is the stage where efforts are made to support and maintain the behavioral gains that have been made. This period is defined as extending from 6 months after the beginning of the action stage onward. Consolidating gains, stabilizing behavior changes, and preventing relapse are considered the hallmarks of this stage.

The stages-of-change model provides motivational interviewing with a conceptual road map for assessing both a client's present position and his or her course. Rather than waiting for the "right" moment or the "window of opportunity" to act, motivational interviewing meets the client wherever he or she is with "stage-appropriate" strategies. For example, a practitioner of motivational interviewing will work increase the perception of risk and problems in a precontemplator, but will assist a client in the preparation stage with specific strategies to commence action. Client resistance is utilized as feedback indicating that the practitioner is too far ahead of the client along the motivational continuum. When this is the case, the practitioner's task is to back up and meet the client where he or she is, then begin moving forward again. Table 3.1 describes the primary motivational tasks with which a therapist helps a client move through the various stages of change (Miller & Rollnick, 1991).

In our experience, few students voluntarily consult with health care providers to discuss potential hazards associated with their use of alcohol. Students are often curious about alcohol effects and information about drinking. However, like drinkers in other age groups across the lifespan, few students with hazardous drinking patterns are ready for or interested in changing these patterns at the start of a preventive intervention. For many, just thinking about changing their drinking may be something they do for the first time in the context of BASICS. Practitioners working with high-risk college drinkers can expect to encounter a great deal of resistance and ambivalence to change in their efforts to change the students' drinking behavior. Motivational interviewing provides both a conceptual treatment frame and specific strategies to understand and effectively work with resistance.

From a motivational interviewing perspective, the practitioner's primary objective in working with a precontemplative student is to increase awareness of the ways in which his or her drinking may be hazardous and/or problematic. This may take the form of comparing the number and range of negative consequences a student experiences as a result of binge drinking to college norms for such consequences. It may also include figuring out the number of hours the student spends drinking or recovering from drinking, or the monthly cost of the alcohol needed to maintain the current pattern of

TABLE 3.1. Therapist Motivational Tasks

Client's stage of readiness	Therapist's motivational tasks
Precontemplation	Raise doubt; increase the client's perception of risks and problems with current behaviors.
Contemplation	Tip the balance of ambivalence in the direction of change; elicit reasons to change and identify risks of not changing; strengthen client's self-efficacy for changing current behavior.
Preparation	Help the client identify and select the best initial course of action to commence change; reinforce movement in this direction.
Action	Continue to help the client take steps toward change; provide encouragement and positive reinforcement (e.g., praise) for action steps.
Maintenance	Teach client relapse prevention skills.

Note. Adapted from Miller and Rollnick (1991). Copyright 1991 by The Guilford Press. Adapted by permission.

use. Once the student has begun to contemplate the pros and cons of his or her drinking, the next counseling task is to help the student resolve ambivalence. Not only must the student recognize that the benefits to change outweigh the costs of maintaining the status quo; he or she must also **want** to change. The practitioner's primary task is to help "tip the balance" of ambivalence in the direction of change. Through the interviewing process, the practitioner attempts to elicit reasons to change, while also identifying risks of not changing (e.g., more time for studying, which increases the probability of earning higher grades; fear of not getting accepted to graduate school if grades fall; etc.). The practitioner also seeks to increase the client's belief that he or she can make the desired changes.

Students will naturally vary considerably in the extent and nature of their ambivalence. Some factors that may influence the degree of ambivalence are the following: (1) the amount of thinking about alcohol use the student has done prior to commencing with BASICS or after the initial assessment; (2) the extent to which the student has experienced severe or salient negative consequences associated directly with drinking; (3) the length of time the student has experienced such problems; (4) prior efforts to change hazardous drinking behavior; and (5) whether the student has friends or family members who have experienced salient or severe negative consequences from hazardous drinking (e.g., date rape, alcohol overdose, car accident, etc.).

Once ambivalence is adequately addressed and the client is prepared to make concrete changes in his or her behavior, the primary task of the practitioner becomes helping the client select the best route to change. This may include serving as an educational resource for the client as he or she considers different treatment approaches (e.g., abstinence, Alcoholics Anonymous, Rational Recovery, Moderation Management, etc.). In addition, the practitioner provides praise and positive reinforcement as the client takes steps toward action. In the action stage, the practitioner provides further praise for action steps and helps the client continue taking these steps. Once the behavioral goal is in hand (the maintenance stage), the practitioner's primary therapy task becomes helping the client to prevent a relapse.

Consistent with the perspective of harm reduction, motivational interviewing also views any step in the direction of behavior change as a favorable outcome (Rollnick, Heather, & Bell, 1992). Although it is preferable for a precontemplative student to decide to commence safer drinking practices following the brief intervention, helping this student recognize the ways in which his or her drinking pattern is hazardous is itself viewed as a successful outcome. Assisting a student to resolve ambivalence about changing his or her pattern of drinking also constitutes a success for the motivational interviewing therapist. From this perspective, the client is presumed to have the necessary "stuff" to continue in the direction of behavior change, once the problem has been identified and the ambivalence conflict resolved. Once these motivational barriers are removed, motivational interviewing assumes that the client will persist in the direction of changing his or her behavior well after the brief intervention or treatment phase.

Cognitive-Behavioral Approach to High-Risk Behaviors

Like Marlatt and Gordon's (1985) relapse prevention, BASICS takes a cognitive-behavioral approach to addressing a biopsychosocial problem—namely, high-risk drinking among college students. Whereas relapse prevention focuses primarily on maintenance of treatment gains, BASICS focuses on indicated prevention (or, in the scheme illustrated in Figure 3.2, secondary prevention). Problems associated with heavy drinking are understood as problems to be solved. Behaviors include all physical overt and covert actions and movements; thinking, problem solving, perceiving, imagining, writing, speaking, gesturing, and observing; and all physiological behaviors, such as blushing, crying, and heart palpitations (Linehan, 1993). The essence of cognitive-behavioral therapy is (1) identifying the behavior(s) to change, and (2) understanding the functional relationship between the individual's behaviors and the context in which the behaviors are embedded.

The original relapse prevention model focuses on strategy building in three areas: (1) anticipating lapses and relapses, and preventing them from occurring; (2) coping effectively with a lapse or relapse, so as to minimize its negative consequences and outcome, and to maximize learning from the experience; and (3) reducing global health risks and replacing lifestyle imbalance with balance and moderation. The cognitive-behavioral approach teaches a client how to anticipate, identify, and manage high-risk situations, while also preparing for the future by striving for lifestyle balance; it seeks to outfit the client with the necessary behavioral "tools" to use whenever and wherever signs of trouble appear, rather than encouraging the client to rely on "willpower" alone to maintain behavioral changes.

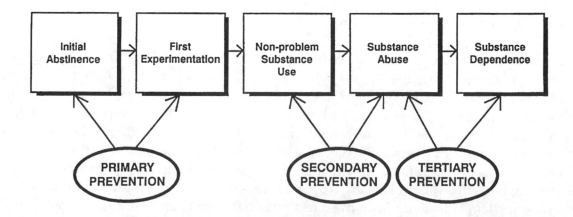

FIGURE 3.2. Stages of development of substance abuse and dependence: Prevention strategies.

Defined broadly, a **high-risk situation** is one in which the individual's sense of perceived control is threatened. A high-risk situation can be an environmental occurrence, an interpersonal interaction, or an internal state that triggers a person to engage in the unwanted behavior. If the person copes effectively in the high-risk situation, the individual will experience an increase in **self-efficacy,** or the belief that he or she can respond successfully to other high-risk situations in the future and maintain the goal. Such an experience decreases the probability of a future relapse. However, if a person is not able to generate an effective coping response, he or she may experience an increase in passivity, helplessness, and a sense of being out of control. These circumstances function to increase the probability that coping skills will not be used and that a slip or relapse will occur.

As a first step, relapse prevention seeks to help the client identify the circumstances when his or her sense of control over the situation is threatened. Once identified, the therapist can then focus on problem-solving and skill-building activities designed to bolster coping in these situations. Should a slip occur, the client is taught specific skills to use to prevent further "slippage." This includes a discussion of the **goal violation effect** (also referred to as the **abstinence violation effect** when the goal is abstinence). The goal violation effect consists of the cognitive and affective responses experienced by the individual following a slip or lapse, such as frustration, feeling demoralized, or giving up on efforts to change. Preparing the client for such reactions includes developing a set of skills to combat these experiences, should the client violate his or her goal.

The central principles of cognitive-behavioral relapse prevention are adapted to the arena of prevention in BASICS. These adapted principles are summarized below.

Identifying High-Risk Drinking Situations

Few young adults consider their drinking risky or excessive and few attempt to regulate or "manage" their drinking. The first task is to increase a student's awareness of individual drinking behavior and to identify particular situational factors that contribute to hazardous consumption. Self-monitoring, as described later in this manual, is one behavioral technique used to increase the student's awareness of his or her drinking while identifying specific circumstances that correspond with heavy drinking occasions. Another approach is to ask the student to identify the settings where he or she is likely to drink in a hazardous fashion. Although patterns of drinking vary widely from student to student, individual's patterns are relatively consistent. For example, sorority women at the University of Washington typically drink alcohol at parties (weekend nights), during weeknight gatherings between brother and sister fraternities and sororities in the Greek system, and at formal dances. Because alcohol is not allowed in sororities on campus, but is allowed in certain areas in fraternities, sorority women typically drink at fraternities. Students are often able to describe their general drinking habits, but tend to have greater difficulty discerning more subtle situational factors (e.g., who, what, where, when). In BASICS, students are helped to identify these factors.

Providing Accurate Information about Alcohol

Although many students are familiar with the potential long-term hazards of heavy drinking, few consider more proximal negative drinking outcomes (e.g., alcohol overdose, alcohol-related lethal accident, etc.). Students are provided with information about alcohol's short-term negative consequences, so that they will be adequately prepared to discuss ways to drink more safely. As part of BASICS, students learn basic facts about alcohol, such as how to calculate their approximate blood alcohol level (BAL), what constitutes a standard drink, how alcohol is metabolized, what tolerance is, how men and women differ in their metabolizing of alcohol, and what the drinking norms are for college students and for the general population across the lifespan. (Much of this information is provided for readers themselves later in this chapter.)

Identifying Personal Risk Factors

Personal factors that may contribute to the risk of developing alcohol-related problems are identified next. Individual factors include a positive family history of alcohol problems, a history of conduct disorder or behavioral dyscontrol, or a history of heavy drinking and alcohol-related consequences. Students receive this feedback primarily to broaden their understanding of their personal risks and to highlight the less obvious factors that contribute to present or future problems with alcohol. In addition, it enables a practitioner to recommend and refer those for whom abstinence is indicated.

Challenging of Myths and Positive Alcohol Expectancies

Students are encouraged to examine their beliefs about what they expect to experience or feel when drinking. Students quite commonly believe that the pharmacological properties of alcohol contribute to improved social functioning, including feeling more relaxed, socially outgoing, friendly, and sexually attractive. Not surprisingly, these positive alcohol expectancies often provide the incentive to drink. In addition, many young drinkers also believe that the pleasure they expect to derive from drinking is commensurate to the amount they consume. The false belief that "more is better" further encourages heavy drinking. These beliefs and expectancies are challenged through several techniques, including self-monitoring and information about placebo effects.

Establishing More Appropriate and Safer Drinking Goals

Moderation goals are encouraged for persons choosing to drink. **Moderation** is defined as drinking alcohol in a way that avoids intoxication and alcohol-related problems. Drinking limits are encouraged (e.g., keeping the BAL at 0.055% or below). We have found that few students give much thought to moderation or limits. Few students are able to specify the criteria they use to determine when they have had enough to drink.

Managing High-Risk Drinking Situations

Specific cognitive and behavioral strategies to initiate and maintain safer drinking limits are then taught and practiced through role play and homework. Cognitive strategies include reminding oneself of the established goal (particularly before a drinking function) and using imagery and self-talk to overcome urges to exceed the goal. Behavioral techniques include avoiding high-risk drinking situations, practicing assertive behaviors (e.g., drink refusal), and engaging in behavioral alternatives (e.g., alternating alcoholic with nonalcoholic drinks, spacing drinks, consuming drinks with lower alcohol content).

Learning from Mistakes

Mistakes often occur when an individual trying to change an old behavior. Unfortunately, mistakes often result in negative and counterproductive feelings (e.g., discouragement, guilt, embarrassment, and sometimes depression), which can compromise a person's motivation and interest in continuing to work toward behavior change. As noted earlier, in the relapse prevention literature this set of responses is known as the **goal violation effect,** and is illustrated by the following sentences: "What's the point? I gave my all; I just can't do it!" or "Oh, well. I guess this just isn't the time to be making these changes." To avoid this effect, slips or lapses in pursing the target behavior are reframed as opportunities for the student to learn more about high-risk situations and to fine-tune his or her repertoire of more effective coping responses. When the goal is moderation, a lapse constitutes drinking beyond the set limit of drinks, drinking to intoxication, or drinking in a way that results in problems (e.g., fights, arguments, or driving while intoxicated).

Increasing Self-Efficacy

Using the self-efficacy theory of Albert Bandura (1977), we attempt to help students enhance their belief in their own ability to make and maintain healthy changes in their consumption of drinking. In the field of addictive behaviors, different types of self-efficacy exist for different stages of the problem. **Resistance self-efficacy** (the ability to resist pressure to drink or refuse drugs in the first place; Hays & Ellickson, 1990) and **harm reduction self-efficacy** (one's perceived ability to experiment with or use drugs in a way that reduces harmful consequences; Marlatt et al., 1993) are two types applicable to primary and secondary prevention efforts, respectively. Peer influence plays a primary role in the initiation of drug use in adolescents, but is often moderated by beliefs in one's ability to resist pressure to use drugs (Stacy, Sussman, Dent, Burton, & Flay, 1992). A similar moderating effect is hypothesized to occur for students who have already initiated use of alcohol.

Attaining Lifestyle Balance

Finally, BASICS participants are encouraged to establish and maintain a balanced lifestyle. This is achieved by balancing "shoulds" (things they feel they have to do) with "wants" (things they do for themselves to obtain pleasure), and by replacing rigid and maladaptive behavior patterns with "positive addictions" (Glasser, 1976), such as aerobic exercise, meditation, or other relaxation techniques. This is particularly relevant for students before midterm and final examinations, and around the deadlines for term papers. Many students sequester themselves in quiet places, study for hours on end, and deprive themselves of sleep and fun—all in the name of pushing hard for peak performance. Once the goals are met and the tests are taken, heavy partying becomes a way of "rewarding" themselves for working hard. Helping such a student balance his or her lifestyle can often include helping the student to organize time more efficiently throughout the quarter or semester, in order to prevent "binge studying," "all-nighters," and the concomitant postevent partying. It can also include helping the student survive the academic hurdles in a more humane and saner fashion by balancing productive studying hours with rest and fun, so as to avoid the deprivation-driven desire to "party."

Integrating Motivational Interviewing and Cognitive-Behavioral Skills Training

Like many other cognitive-behavioral treatments, BASICS is based on a model that combines capability deficit and motivational aspects. In other words, it assumes (1) that students lack information and skills that facilitate moderate drinking, and (2) that they have motivational deficits in making use of the information and resources they do have. It is for this reason that BASICS draws heavily from both cognitive-behavioral skills training and motivational interviewing. We see this integration of strategies to build skills and enhance motivation as consistent with many behavior therapies, and as necessary and essential in BASICS.

Although they are commonly integrated in actual clinical practice, motivational interviewing and skills training are often described in controlled clinical trials of treatment conditions in ways that imply diametrical opposition and mutual exclusion (Kadden et al., 1994; Miller et al., 1992). Motivational interviewing is offered as an intervention for managing client resistance and ambivalence toward change, which are of particular importance for clients in the precontemplative and contemplative stages of change. The assumption behind skills training is that a state of readiness for change exists, but that the individual lacks the skills to make the desired change. In contrast to skills training, for example, a motivational interviewing approach does not teach the client ways to change his or her behavior; no role plays, practice and feedback sessions, modeling, or problem-solving sessions are conducted in motivational interviewing. Instead, the client is viewed as being capable of and responsible for developing his or her own methods for change. Motivational interviewing seeks both to elicit and to develop the client's own intrinsic motivation. Goals and specific skills used to make changes come from the client (once he or she is ready to make changes). Skills training, in contrast, tends to assume motivational readiness on the part of the client, and seeks to identify and correct ineffective cognitive and behavioral coping strategies. Miller and Rollnick (1991) emphasize this dichotomy as shown in Table 3.2.

In reality, motivational enhancement strategies (including motivational interviewing) and cognitive-behavioral skills training are commonly utilized in tandem, because both are typically required: motivation to provide the will, and skills training to provide the way. Perhaps the marks of a truly outstanding clinician are knowing when to focus on which, and moving quickly and gracefully between the two in a moment-by-moment fashion.

BASIC INFORMATION ABOUT ALCOHOL

General information about alcohol is embedded throughout the second session of BASICS. Although the primary aim of the initial session is to assess the student's pattern of alcohol use and personal risk factors, an opportunity may also arise during this first meeting to educate the student about alcohol. We provide a fuller discussion later in the manual of how to provide students with this information, in addition to some cautionary notes. For now, it is important to note that the provision of this information must be well timed. As a general rule, we recommend that the information provided should "fit" into the context of the natural discussion—in other words, that its introduction should be relevant to the topic at hand and meaningful to the student.

TABLE 3.2. Primary Differences between Motivational Interviewing and Skills Training

Skills training approach	Motivational interviewing approach
Assumes that the client is motivated; no direct strategies are used for building motivation.	Employs specific principles and strategies for building client's motivation for change.
Seeks to identify and modify maladaptive cognitions.	Explores and reflects client's perceptions without labeling or "correcting" them.
Prescribes specific coping strategies.	Elicits possible change strategies from the client.
Teaches coping behaviors through instruction, modeling, direct practice, and feedback.	Responsibility for change methods is left with the client; no training, modeling, or practice is employed.
Specific problem-solving strategies are taught.	Natural problem-solving processes are elicited from the client.

Note. Adapted from Miller and Rollnick (1991). Copyright 1991 by The Guilford Press. Adapted by permission.

Positive Alcohol Expectancies

The following questions about alcohol expectancies are usually raised with students:

- To what extent are the effects we experience after drinking alcohol psychological versus pharmacological in nature?

- Is it possible to feel "buzzed," light-headed, and "tipsy" from tonic water alone?

- Can our beliefs about how alcohol effects us actually contribute to experiencing that effect after drinking? How much is our experience of alcohol's effects "all in our heads"?

Students commonly believe, for example, that the pharmacological aspects of alcohol are responsible for their experience of social and sexual disinhibition. If this is true, the job of encouraging some students to moderate their alcohol use becomes a more complex "sell." If, however, psychological factors are indeed as important as (and in some cases more important than) the actual pharmacological factors, the preventive intervention can focus on psychological strategies or behaviors to achieve the same effect.

A series of experiments conducted in the 1970s and 1980s (for reviews, see Marlatt & Rohsenow, 1980; Hull & Bond, 1986) sought to untangle the extent to which a person's experience after drinking alcohol is psychological versus pharmacological, and the extent to which a person's expectations of what will happen after drinking influence the person's actual experience after drinking. These studies demonstrated that much of the postdrinking experience is based on expectancy effects, or what a person expects to feel or experience. To control for psychological and pharmacological effects, a 2 × 2 balanced-placebo design was utilized in this research. That is, the kind of beverage (alcohol vs. tonic water) was varied by what subjects were told they would receive (expected alcohol vs. expected tonic). As illustrated in Figure 3.3, one group expected to get alcohol and did receive alcohol; another expected tonic water and received tonic water; a third expected alcohol, but instead received tonic water laced with a drop of rum extract (placebo condition); the fourth expected tonic water, but instead received vodka (spiked-drink condition).

The results from these balanced-placebo studies are summarized in Table 3.3. Generally, both women and men experienced a disinhibiting effect from the belief that they had consumed even mild amounts of alcohol. Interestingly, whereas men generally became less socially anxious when they believed they had consumed alcohol, women reported more social anxiety in the same condition. Men typically perceived greater sexual arousal when they believed they had consumed alcohol; however, physiological sexual response was actually dampened in both women and men. Finally, alcohol expectancies appeared to be particularly salient for men in their experience of aggression, with aggression being associated primarily with the belief that they had consumed alcohol in moderate doses.

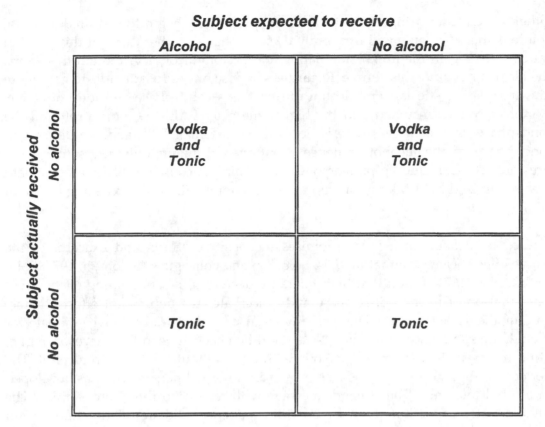

FIGURE 3.3. The 2 × 2 balanced-placebo design.

In addition to the balanced-placebo studies on alcohol expectancies, studies have been conducted using self-report questionnaires to assess an individual's alcohol expectancies, in addition to the salience of these expectancies (Fromme, Stroot, & Kaplan, 1993; Leigh, 1989). The results of these studies support those of the balanced-placebo research.

Debunking the Myth That "More Is Better": The Biphasic Response

As a person consumes alcohol in low to moderate amounts and as his or her BAL is ascending (i.e., usually during the initial phase of drinking), alcohol at first produces mild arousal, experienced as excitement, increased energy, and increased confidence. This is illustrated in Figure 3.4 by the initial rise on the curves on the "feeling scale." Over time, however, the effects became more depressant in nature and may be experienced as fatigue, "slowing down," and lack of coordination. Again, the initial positive phase is associated with low but rising BALs; in contrast, the negative phase that follows is associated more with falling BALs, regardless of whether a person's peak BAL is high or low (although the drop is sharper when the peak is higher; see Figure 3.4).

In other words, after drinking for a while, people usually begin to feel tired and lose that initial "high." People will frequently decide to have another drink at this point in an attempt to regain the initial stimulating effects from alcohol. Although this seems plausible, it's not quite this simple. Regardless of dose or desire, attempts to gain more of the stimulating effects from alcohol during this second phase are nonproductive. The more alcohol consumed and the higher the peak BAL, the more profound the second phase. In this sense, there is no escaping a falling BAL and the depressant second phase of the alcohol response. Continued drinking only leads to greater depressant effects, including passing out or becoming unconscious. The second phase can be minimized by drinking low to moderate amounts (i.e., not exceeding a BAL of 0.06%).

Tolerance to alcohol further compromises the positive effects and exacerbates the negative effects. Using animal models, Solomon and colleagues (Solomon, 1977; Solomon & Corbit, 1974) found that high tolerance decreases the stimulating effects from alcohol that occur in the initial phase and exacerbates the depressant effects characteristic of the second phase. These findings can provide an additional rationale for reducing one's tolerance to alcohol. Note the difference between the curves in Figure 3.4 that represent this effect for persons with and without tolerance to alcohol. The lower curve displays the biphasic response to alcohol for a person who has developed high alcohol tolerance. The primary message with respect to this point is this: "The more and faster you drink, the **less** you will experience mild stimulating effects, and the **more** you will feel depressant effects."

TABLE 3.3. Summary of Results from Balanced-Placebo Research

Men	Women
Social anxiety	
Men became less anxious in social situations when they believed they had had alcohol.	Women became more anxious in social situations when they believed they had had alcohol.
Aggression	
Men became more aggressive when they were drinking only tonic water, but believed their drink contained alcohol.	
Men became relatively less aggressive then they thought they were drinking tonic water, but their drink actually contained alcohol.	
Sexual arousal	
Men perceived themselves as more sexually aroused when they believed their drink contained alcohol, in the absence of objective physiological arousal.	Women became less sexually aroused when drinking alcohol.

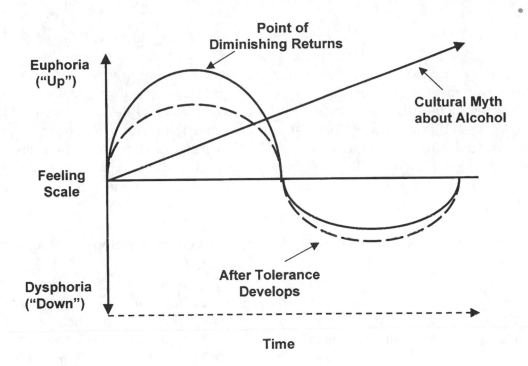

FIGURE 3.4. The biphasic response to alcohol.

Many college students perceive heavy drinking as highly pleasurable. Students quite commonly associate drinking large quantities of alcohol with "partying" and other enjoyable bonding activities, such as dancing, playing, and meeting dating partners. Students seldom mention the negative side effects associated with heavy drinking. There are several possible explanations for this phenomenon. It may be that the positive experiences are more salient than the negative experiences. The social context where heavy drinking occurs may be so positive that the experience of negative physical or psychological effects (e.g., feeling physically drained or ill the next morning, the sense of having made a fool of oneself) pales in comparison. In a sense, therefore, the student may be more likely to remember the pleasurable aspects have associated with heavy alcohol use than the negative consequences. During the second session of BASICS, the therapist attempts to increase the client's awareness of these negative short-term effects by linking the "morning-after" hangover and other negative effects to the drinking behavior that occurred the night before. This is done by exploring the client's experiences to elucidate both the costs and benefits of heavy drinking. In bridging the enjoyable drinking occasion to the hangover the next day, the therapist might ask, "How did you feel the next morning?"

Alcohol Myopia

Students also learn about how and why alcohol can affect the same person differently from one time to the next—perhaps sometimes making a person hostile and aggressive, and at other times friendly and warm. Steele and Josephs (1990) have described a process in which alcohol intoxication creates a kind of cognitive nearsightedness, or "myopia"; that is, it limits information processing and abstract reasoning to simple, immediate, and concrete cues. For example, persons typically process information in a quick and efficient manner, drawing on many different bits of information. Meaning is inferred through assimilating a large body of both subtle and obvious cues. Laboratory studies on alcohol have shown that intoxication impairs cognitive processes by reducing the range of what people perceive and process. In a fashion similar to visual myopia, the perceptions and emotions of a person under the influence of alcohol are restricted to immediate and obvious cues; peripheral and subtle cues are missed.

We sometimes tell students an illustrative story based on one developed by Steele and Josephs (1990) to make this point:

> "Imagine that you have just had a dispute with a teacher over receiving a low grade. The instructor has a reputation for unfair exams and grading practices, and after attempting to reason with him after class, you have no recourse but to accept the low grade. You leave his office playing it cool, but inside you are still outraged. Later that evening, you attend your friend's party, hoping to unwind. You approach the dance floor and accidentally bump into someone standing behind you. As you turn to apologize, you realize you've just run into your instructor. Under any circumstances, his presence would bring forth a desire to impulsively tell him off. If you are sober, you will automatically quickly recognize that this would undoubtedly make matters worse between you and the instructor, not to mention outrage your friend and cause you embarrassment. So you refrain, greet him, and apologize instead. Now suppose that you are intoxicated and that alcohol myopia has reduced your processing abilities to immediate and short-sighted reactions. Myopia limits your ability to think through the negative consequences that could follow from expressing your anger. As a result, you tell him off. Before you know it, a scene develops; your friend sneers at you and asks that you leave; and you fail the course miserably."

Whether a practitioner uses the story above or elicits illustrative examples from a student, the discussion of alcohol myopia should also highlight how alcohol can cause the same person to feel one way on one occasion and the opposite on another by becoming "locked" into whatever is most prominent and salient in the surroundings, in how the person feels (e.g., bored, sad, angry, etc.), or both.

Differential Risks for Women and Men

In recent years, growing attention has been paid to gender differences in the field of alcohol studies as more has become known about differences between women and men in alcohol metabolism and other effects. Our aim in this section is to highlight some of the main differences we believe are important in delivering BASICS.

Gender Differences in Alcohol Intake and Metabolism

Over two decades ago, researchers Ben and Marilyn Jones (Jones & Jones, 1976) published the first laboratory results showing a differential dose effect of alcohol for men and women. In these early studies, women obtained significantly higher BALs than men when administered the same dose of alcohol (adjusted for body weight). In light of the usual weight differences between men and women, Jones and Jones warned that a woman matching drinks with a male counterpart is likely to become twice as intoxicated. Figure 3.5 illustrates the difference in approximate BAL between a man and a woman who both weigh 140 pounds after consuming five standard drinks in 2 hours. Although the two are the same weight, his approximate BAL is estimated at 0.101% and hers at 0.128%. When the usual weight differences between college-age women and men are taken into consideration, the gender gap in estimated BALs widens further. A typical college-age male weighs approximately 180 pounds, while a college-age female weighs on average 130 pounds. In the same drinking scenario described above, his BAL would be estimated at 0.072%, while hers would be nearly double, at 0.134%—considerably over the Washington State legal driving limit of 0.10%. Several factors account for these gender differences in degree of intoxication:

1. *Difference in body water content between women and men.* Whereas the total body weight of men is composed of 55–65% water, women's total body weight is composed of 45–55% water. Hence alcohol becomes more diluted in men than in women.

2. *Difference in levels of gastric alcohol dehydrogenase between women and men.* Alcohol dehydrogenase, a stomach enzyme that aids in metabolism of alcohol, is significantly higher in men than in women. Frezza et al. (1990) found that gastric alcohol dehydrogenase activities were 70–80% higher in a sample of nonalcoholic men than in a sample of nonalcoholic women. These differences in first-pass metabolism appear to make women more vulnerable than men to the development of liver cirrhosis, brain damage, and other health conditions resulting from chronic alcohol abuse (National Institute on Alcohol Abuse and Alcoholism [NIAAA], 1993; Lieber, 1994).

3. *Hormonal changes in women.* Hormonal changes in women can also affect BALs. Specifically, 1 week prior to menstruating, women maintain the peak degree of intoxication for longer periods of time than menstruating or postmenstruating women do. A similar pattern of extended peak intoxication was found in women using oral contraceptives. Jones and Jones (1976) attributed this prolonged peak to an increase in estrogen, which is thought to slow alcohol metabolism.

Despite empirically derived knowledge of gender differences in the field of alcohol studies, clinical standards for assessing and treating alcohol problems often fail to account for these differences. Until recently, alcohol research involving animals and humans has relied primarily on male samples (NIAAA, 1992). Furthermore, comparisons of drinking patterns across gender have also ignored gender differences in alcohol

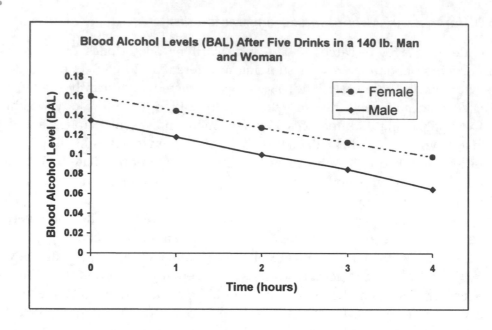

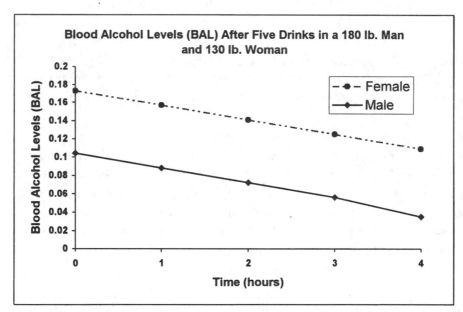

FIGURE 3.5. Comparison of different BALs after five drinks in a 140-pound man and woman and in a 180-pound man and 130-pound woman.

intake and alcohol metabolism, and have instead relied on self-report "unisex" surveys (Dimeff, Baer, & Marlatt, 1994). Though these surveys are considered reliable, their failure to account for weight and sex differences compromises their validity. Not surprisingly, such studies have consistently found lower rates of alcohol use by women (except for lesbian samples) across drinking measures, resulting in a belief that most women are at lower risk for health problems from alcohol (Engs & Hanson, 1990; Perkins, 1992; Wechsler & Isaac, 1992; Wechsler, Davenport, et al., 1994).

TABLE 3.4. Means and Standard Deviations for Conventional and Corrected Drinking Measures

| | Men | | Women | | |
	M	*SD*	*M*	*SD*	*F*
Peak quantity consumed	3.74	1.47	2.96	1.35	22.67**
Typical quantity consumed	2.23	1.5	1.6	1.04	17.74**
Total drinks per week	12.14	11.68	6.95	5.91	24.09**
Peak BAL	0.06%	0.05%	0.06%	0.06%	1.97
Average BAL	0.05%	0.04%	0.06%	0.04%	2.87
Typical frequency	2.75	1.09	2.42	1.0	6.94*

Note. For the assessment of drinking frequency, response options and associated labels were as follows: 0 (less than once a month), 1 (about once a month), 2 (two or three times a month), 3 (once or twice a week), 4 (three or four times a week), and 5 (nearly every day or every day). Assessment of typical drinking quantity and most recent peak consumption were recorded using the following response options and associated labels: 0 (no drinks), 1 (one or two drinks), 2 (three or four drinks), 3 (five or six drinks), 4 (seven or eight drinks), and 5 (more than eight drinks). From Dimeff, Baer, and Marlatt (1994).

$^*p < .01.$ $^{**}p < .001.$

We were interested in examining the gender differences in alcohol consumed by participants in our research project. To assess these differences, we used both conventional quantity measures and gender-sensitive measures that factor in physiological and weight differences (Dimeff et al., 1994).[1] We predicted that the conventional quantity measures would show significantly higher rates of drinking among men than among women, but that these differences would disappear when the data were reanalyzed with a multidimensional measure correcting for weight and gender. When the conventional measures were employed, men **appeared** to drink significantly more than women across all measures, including peak quantity consumed, frequency of use, and total drinks consumed per week (see Table 3.4). On the basis of these statistical findings, it would appear that the college men in our sample typically consumed nearly twice as much alcohol per week as the women did. Once the data were reanalyzed with measures such as a typical week's peak BAL adjusted for gender and weight, the differences in group averages were no longer above chance levels. Although no differences in quantity emerged, the men in our sample reported drinking more frequently than women, which may indeed increase the likelihood of problems.

Increased Risk of Sexual Assault and/or Rape

In 1987, Koss et al. first published their findings from their extensive nationwide study of rape on campus, involving 6,159 students from 32 colleges and universities. Their findings included the following:

---

[1] In the gender-sensitive assessment, students reported the typical number of drinks they consumed on each day of the week in the past month. In addition, they were asked to indicate the typical number of hours spent consuming alcoholic beverages for each day of the week. BAL estimates were then calculated for each day, according to a formula developed by Matthews and Miller (1979).

- One in four women participated in the study reported being a victim of either rape or attempted rape.

- Of these, 84% knew their attackers, and 57% of the rapes occurred in the context of a date.

- Twelve percent of the men reported committing acts that met the legal definition of rape or attempted rape.

- Seventy-five percent of the men and 55% of the women reported having used alcohol or other drugs prior to the sexual assault.

Other studies of acquaintance rape have also found substantial rates of alcohol use by the victim and/or the perpetrator. Muehlenhard and Linton (1987) reported these findings:

- Twenty-six percent of the college men the surveyed reported committing sexual assault.

- Twenty-one percent of the women victims were intoxicated at the time of the assault.

- Twenty-nine percent of the men and 32% of the women described being "mildly buzzed" at the time of the sexual assault.

In recent survey research conducted at another large urban university, 26% of 814 males ranging in age from 18 to 59 reported perpetrating sexual assault (Abbey, McAuslan, & Ross, 1998). Of 1,160 undergraduate women surveyed, over half reported experiencing some form of sexual assault; of these, nearly half involved use of alcohol either by the man, woman, or both (Abbey, Ross, McDuffie, & McAuslan, 1996a).

How and to what extent does alcohol serve as a risk factor for rape and attempted rape, and what are the implications for rape prevention? These are important questions that have received greater attention in recent years. Given that women in their early 20s are at three times greater risk for sexual victimization than women in other age groups, this topic is particularly relevant in the context of preventing binge drinking among college students. From her extensive review of the research literature, Antonia Abbey (1991) and her colleagues (Abbey, McAuslan, & Ross, 1998; Abbey et al., 1996b) points to several explanations for the relationship between alcohol use and sexual aggression:

1. *Men's expectancies about alcohol effects.* Men often expect to feel more sexual, powerful, and aggressive after drinking alcohol (Brown, Goldman, Inn, & Anderson, 1980). We do not need to look any further than alcohol advertisements directed at college-age men to understand the ways which these outcome expectancies are formed and the power of the imagery evoked. Abbey (1991) notes, "The *belief* that one has consumed alcohol does . . . produce greater physiological and psychological sexual

arousal. Men who think they have been drinking alcohol feel sexually aroused and are more responsive to erotic stimuli, including rape scenarios" (p. 166; emphasis in original).

2. *Men's misperceptions of sexual intent.* Abbey further notes that men are more likely than women to interpret verbal and nonverbal cues as indicators of a woman's interest in having sex with a man. Several studies have demonstrated that college men perceive women as being more seductive and promiscuous, and more interested in having sex, than women perceive themselves as being (Abbey, 1982, 1987; Abbey & Melby, 1986). Abbey (1991) interprets the results of these studies as evidence that "men view the world in a more sexualized manner than women do and, consequently, are more likely than women to interpret ambiguous cues as evidence of sexual intent" (p. 166), and she adds that women are socialized to assume a gatekeeper's role while men pursue. In this context, the socialized script for women involves both flirting in both direct and indirect ways, and resisting advances so as not to appear "loose" or "easy." This script may make it more easy for a man to ignore a woman's "no" and force sex on her against her will.

Adding alcohol to the equation can further increase the probability that misperceptions of sexual intent can take place. Recall the discussion of alcohol myopia, above: Alcohol intoxication can result in a narrowing of the ability to process and analyze complex stimuli from the environment. Particularly in the context of heavy drinking, an intoxicated man may be more likely to interpret ambiguous cues in a way that is consistent with his own feeling state or desires.

3. *Alcohol consumption as a justification for men's sexual violence.* College men, according to Abbey, may drink purposely to experience the positive outcomes they expect from drinking—namely, a sense of disinhibition, increased sexual ease, and power. The next day, however, they "write off," discount, or brag about whatever socially unacceptable acts they committed the night before, using alcohol in this sense as an excuse.

4. *Alcohol's effects on women's ability to send and receive cues.* Intoxicated women are more vulnerable to acts of sexual aggression, as alcohol myopia reduces a drinking woman's ability to recognize subtle and complex signals that would otherwise alert her to her partner's sexual intent or her risk for sexual assault. Because alcohol myopia narrows attention and reduces inferential processing, a woman may not be able to "see" that "her friendly behavior is being perceived as seduction" (Abbey, 1991, p. 167). This is particularly important, given that men are more likely to interpret friendly behavior by women in a dating context as an indication of sexual interest, as noted above.

5. *Alcohol's effect on women's ability to resist sexual assault.* A number of studies have demonstrated that a woman's ability to verbally and physically resist a sexual assault becomes impaired as a function of her degree of intoxication, because of the resulting

cognitive and physical impairment (Koss & Dinero, 1989; Golding, Siegel, Sorenson, Burnam, & Stein, 1989).

6. *Stereotypes about women who consume alcohol.* Research by George and colleagues (George, Gournic, & McAffee, 1988; George, Cue, Lopez, & Crowe-Leif, 1995; George & Marlatt, 1986) has shown that college students typically perceive a woman drinking alcohol as (a) more sexually disinhibited, (b) more likely to enjoy being the recipient of seduction, and (c) more willing to engage in foreplay and sexual intercourse than a woman drinking a soft drink. Men were also found to be more likely to initiate sexual activity with a drinking woman than with a nondrinker, because of expectations about the sexual receptivity of the female drinker. This may explain why some men purposely attempt to intoxicate a woman (e.g., buying drinks, encouraging participation in drinking games) to increase her vulnerability.

Increased Risk for Disordered Eating

The incidence of eating disorders among college women range from 4.4% (Stangler & Printz, 1980) to 10% (Rand & Kuldau, 1992). A number of studies have documented a significant relationship between disordered eating (defined as patterns of eating or behaviors related to eating that may not meet diagnostic criteria for an eating disorder, but are nonetheless harmful from a health perspective) and alcohol abuse in college women (Krahn, 1991; Yeary & Heck, 1989). In one survey of lifestyle behaviors of 200 randomly selected college women, 19.7% of the participants reported self-induced vomiting (Meilman, von Hippel, & Gaylor, 1991). Three distinct kinds of purgers were identified in this study: those who purged following consumption of alcohol ("drinking purgers"), those who purged following consumption of food ("eating purgers"), and those who purged following either consumption of food or alcohol. Interestingly, the rate of purging after drinking alcohol (7.4%) was considerably higher than that after eating (4.7%), but comparable to the rate of purging after food or alcohol (7.4%). Place of residence predicted eating purgers in this sample, where 72.2% of the nonfreshman women resided in sororities (freshmen were excluded from the analysis, because policy at the university where this survey was conducted prohibits students from living in the Greek system their first year). Although differences in average weekly alcohol consumption between high-frequency eating purgers (22.3 drinks per week) and the remaining sample (17.2 drinks per week) were not statistically significant, significant differences did emerge with respect to the peak quantity consumed in an average week, with eating purgers averaging 36.5 drinks per heavy-drinking week, compared to 24.5 drinks for the remaining sample.

Young women especially women of European descent, are under enormous pressure to be thin (le Grange, Telch, & Tibbs, 1998). Thinness and conventions for female attractiveness are often nearly synonymous terms. In the context of our own research in the Greek system, sorority women have occasionally told us that it is not uncommon to go through a "hazing" process, in which older house members use a permanent marker to circle areas of unacceptable body fat on the bodies of new members (Luce, DuBois, Dimeff, Larimer, & Marlatt, 1993). It also appears that increased concern about body image and appearance is greater in houses with "better" social reputations than in other sororities in the Greek system.

Blood Alcohol Effects

Although the effects of drinking at mild to moderate doses are largely psychological, alcohol nonetheless does have real physical effects upon the central nervous system. At high doses, reaction time, motor control, and cognitive processing are impaired, resulting in an increase in risks of accidents and health risks. During the second session of BASICS, students are informed of the kinds of experiences nontolerant people have at different BALs. Students' experiences at various BALs are then compared to the experiences of persons without tolerance in order to assess the students' degree of tolerance, as well as to make the link between their drinking behavior and its physiological impact "real."

Students learn that BAL is the ratio of alcohol to blood in the bloodstream, and is determined by calculating the milligrams of alcohol per 100 milliliters of blood. BAL is usually reported as a percentage (e.g., 0.10% = 1 part alcohol for every 1,000 parts of blood). In Washington and many other states, an individual is legally found to be driving while intoxicated if he or she is driving with a BAL equal to or greater than 0.10%. In some states, the legal limit is set at 0.08%.

The intoxicating effects of alcohol are the results of alcohol's physiological action on the brain. Alcohol's effects are roughly predictable from the amount of alcohol in the bloodstream for students with minimal tolerance. Predicting alcohol's effects in individuals with tolerance is difficult. Table 3.5 indicates the common alcohol effects at different BALs in persons without marked tolerance. (This information is provided in the "tips" sheets we give to students; see Appendix B.) Students with tolerance to alcohol will often report differences between their personal experience at certain BALs and the standard effects for persons without tolerance described during the session. These perceived differences can open the door for discussing issues involving physiological and behavioral tolerance.

Tolerance

Most heavy-drinking college students show some degree of tolerance to alcohol; that is, they require more alcohol (specifically, a higher BAL) to get the same effect. Many students perceive tolerance as beneficial, since they believe that they will remain more in control of their actions at high BALs. Tolerance can be a liability, however. Not only is it financially expensive; it can also cause organ strain and can increase the likelihood of developing long-term health problems, due to the high levels of toxins in the body for extended periods.

TABLE 3.5. Common Alcohol Effects for Persons without Tolerance

BAL	Common alcohol effects
0.02%	Light and moderate drinkers begin to feel some effect.
0.04%	Most people begin to feel relaxed.
0.06%	Judgment is somewhat impaired; people are less able to make rational decisions about their capabilities (e.g., driving).
0.08%	Definite impairment of muscle coordination and driving skills is evident; increased risk of nausea and slurred speech.
0.10%	Clear deterioration of reaction time.
0.15%	Balance and movement are impaired; risk of blackouts, passing out, and accidents increases dramatically.
0.30%	Most people lose consciousness. Central nervous system is substantially depressed; risk of death.

Fortunately, alcohol tolerance is reversible to a large degree; indeed, it can be reversed relatively quickly with brief periods of abstinence or reduced consumption. Many students, intentionally or unintentionally, have already had the experience of reducing their tolerance—often when they move back home during school breaks or summer vacation. A common strategy for reducing tolerance is for a student to set a safer BAL limit (usually suggested not to exceed 0.06%) and a time period (e.g., 2 months) in which not to exceed this limit. Generally, students who actively undertake this project find that drinking less alcohol has some real advantages, including feeling less "hung over" the following day and having more money for other activities.

The Detrimental Effects of Alcohol Intoxication on Sleep, Alertness, and Performance

Students seldom realize that the alcohol they consume during a single evening can compromise their performance for days to come, as a result of the effects of alcohol intoxication on sleep. The extent to which cognitive and physical performance is impaired by sleep deprivation is directly related to the degree to which a person is intoxicated at the time he or she falls asleep. Generally, the more the individual is intoxicated, the more sleep is disrupted. What kinds of changes in sleep can be expected? The following points summarize the effects of acute alcohol intoxication on sleep (Carskadon & Dement, 1989; Kay & Samiuddin, 1988):

- Total sleep time increases during the first half of the night; it decreases, however, during the second half of the night.

- Wakefulness after sleep onset decreases during the first half of the night; it increases, however, during the second half of the night.

- Rapid eye movement (REM) decreases during the first half of the night; REM rebound occurs in later portions of the night, following alcohol metabolism. Greater levels of intoxication may fully suppress REM sleep and prevent rebound until the following night, because of the set metabolism rate of alcohol (approximately one drink per hour).

- Delta sleep decreases.

What effects can a student expect to experience the following day as a result of this alcohol-induced sleep disturbance? From a psychological perspective, it is not uncommon to experience feeling unrested and unrefreshed, groggy and fatigued, and more irritable than usual. Cognitive dampening is also quite common; this is typically experienced as not feeling as "sharp" or "quick" as one usually does. Finally, mental stamina (e.g., the ability to sustain focus and concentration for periods of time) is diminished as well.

The effects of sleep deprivation on physical performance are comparable to the psychological effects just described (Mougin et al., 1989; Radomski, Hart, Goodman, & Plyley, 1992; VanHelder & Radomski, 1989). Physiologically, sleep deprivation results in the suppression of normal levels of prolactin, cortisol, and growth hormone. Oxygen consumption also decreases at maximal workload; in other words, physical endurance performance may be substantially impaired as a result of temporary impairment to the aerobic pathways.

BASICS CLINICAL AIMS, THERAPIST/CLIENT ISSUES, AND FORMAT

Having now reviewed the theoretical foundation for BASICS and equipped our readers with the necessary psychoeducational information we commonly use in our work with college students, we now turn to the "hows" and "whats" of BASICS.

Aims of BASICS

BASICS has been designed as a flexible, affordable, user-friendly, and effective indicated prevention program to reduce hazardous drinking in college students. For maximal flexibility, each session is tailored to the client's own risk factors and circumstances, as well as to the severity of the client's abuse or dependence. Second, to minimize program cost, the intervention can be easily modified to be implemented by a wide variety of care providers with ranges of clinical experience. It is always easier to do more with additional funds and resources. From our perspective, the challenge was to develop a quick and straightforward approach that could be easily adapted for use by professional and nonprofessional staff with college students. Of course, the key issue is effectiveness. We wanted to devise a program that would not only reduce drinking rates and problems directly, but could also promote appropriate utilization of other services if students should continue to drink in a harmful fashion.

Clinical Approach in BASICS

Instead of a didactic approach that accentuates the schism between "professional" and "patient," BASICS employs an interactive approach in which the client is engaged in the process as a partner in learning. In building this working alliance with the student, the therapist might imagine that he or she and the client are examining the information together, and are collaborating on the course of what action (if any) to pursue. Using techniques from motivational interviewing, the therapist attempts to circumvent common traps that can undermine BASICS's success. For example, labeling a young person as "alcoholic" or "having a problem" often elicits defensiveness on the client's part. This often results in the loss of therapist credibility. (Other specific traps to avoid when working with young adults are described in Chapter 6 of this manual.)

Therapist Matching to BASICS

It is generally not necessary for a practitioner using BASICS to have a great deal of experience in treatment of addictive behaviors or cognitive-behavioral approaches to therapy. It is recommended that the individual be familiar and comfortable with basic counseling skills, such as empathetic and active listening, expressing positive regard for the client, and keeping the client's defensiveness and psychological reactance to a minimum. In addition, the practitioner should be able to assume the role of "professional" comfortably. It has been our experience that the process, content, and tone of BASICS are more important than amount of professional training, educational degree, or clinical experience. Thus far, we have not found differences in treatment effectiveness resulting from differences among care providers in degrees, experience, or training. This is consistent with findings by many others (Christensen & Jacobson, 1994).

Practitioners with a high level of confidence in their knowledge of what is best for each client, and a firm conviction that they must actively persuade each client to accept a particular view, may have difficulty adjusting to this nonconfrontational and nonauthoritarian approach. Other practitioner styles that conflict with this approach include an insistence on giving unequivocal directives to change rather than asking questions and heightening ambivalence, and a preference for using expressions such as "You should. . . . "

How Students Are Recruited

Students participating in the research on BASICS volunteered to do so and were under no obligation or requirement to participate. Prior to enrollment at the university, high school seniors who had accepted an offer of admission to the University of Washington were invited to complete questionnaire about their use of alcohol by mail. High risk drinkers were selected from the pool of individuals who had completed the screening and were invited to participate in the Lifestyles Project. (See Chapter 2 for further details.) Study participants were free at any time to withdraw from participation or to decline services rendered as part of the intervention study.

To our knowledge, no studies have been conducted to date on the efficacy of an indicated alcohol prevention program for "mandated" students. We have sought with limited success to conduct such studies, because it is reasonable to assume that differences in effectiveness may emerge when students are ordered to participate in treatment because of a campus alcohol policy violation. In our experience, students required by school administration are extremely reluctant to participate in research that requires collection of data about the very behaviors that have resulted in their need to obtain the professional services of our group. In the absence of clinical data about the effectiveness of BASICS with mandated students, we are simply uncertain whether much is to be gained by using BASICS in this context.

The BASICS Format

In BASICS, a therapist typically meets with a student in two 50-minute appointments. Basic assessment information is gathered during the first session; this will serve as the material for "feedback" during the subsequent session. After (or, less commonly, before) the initial interview, the student is asked to complete a questionnaire packet of self-report measures that provides additional relevant information about lifestyle behaviors and risks; a further 50-minute period is allowed for this. Before leaving the initial session, the student is also given a homework assignment to monitor his or her drinking. The second session is then scheduled in 1–2 weeks; this allows enough time between sessions for the student to obtain a good "sampling" of drinking episodes while monitoring. During the second session, the student receives basic feedback about his or her drinking pattern and risks, as well as basic information about alcohol and its effects. When appropriate, the student also receives tips and advice in how to reduce risks. Additional booster sessions are scheduled as needed.

The Primary Components of Sessions 1 and 2

Table 3.6 summarizes the primary components for each session and what is needed for each. The various components are described in detail in Chapters 4 and 5. We recommend that meetings be conducted in a private, quiet setting, to provide maximal comfort for both the practitioner and the student. Because of the interactive nature of both sessions, we recommend a seating arrangement that allows the practitioner and client to look together at visual aids and graphs. Ideally, chairs should be reasonably close together and turned slightly in toward each other; we recommend against arranging chairs in such a fashion that the practitioner and client are seated directly in front of each other. An additional quiet room with a table and chair may also be needed for the client to complete measures or questionnaires after (or before) the first meeting.

TABLE 3.6. The BASICS Checklist

Session 1

Components	• Structured clinical interview • Self-report questionnaire packet
Required time	• 100 minutes total, 50 minutes for each component
Needed	• Quiet, private room for the clinical interview • Quiet room with table and chair for student to complete self-report questionnaire packet • Structured Clinical Interview Packet (for therapist) • Self-report questionnaire packet, pencil, and eraser (for student) • Monitoring cards and instructions

Session 2

Components	• Feedback and advice
Required time	• Approximately 50 minutes
Needed	• Personalized graphic feedback sheet • Quiet, private room • Personalized BAL chart • Pocket-size laminated personalized BAL chart • "Tips" sheet

CHAPTER 4

The Initial Assessment Interview

Having reviewed the theoretical and practical foundations of BASICS, we now move directly into discussions of the clinical interviews. This chapter focuses entirely on the initial meeting, from orienting the student to the purpose of the brief intervention to thinking through what to ask in the assessment. We also review the measures used during the initial interview, and we preview the measures we have asked students to complete on their own (either before or after this initial meeting) in our research. A full listing of these various measures is provided in Appendix A.

Objectives and Overview of the First Session

Preparing for the First Session

The Actual Meeting
    Rapport Building, Orienting, and Getting an Initial Commitment
    Assessing High-Risk Lifestyle and Health Behaviors
    Wrapping Up the Initial Interview

Self-Report Questionnaire Packet of Lifestyle Measures

Student Feedback about the Assessment Procedures

OBJECTIVES AND OVERVIEW OF THE FIRST SESSION

The primary tasks of the first session are twofold: (1) to gather information about the student's alcohol use and other health behaviors, which will provide the clinical data for the second session; and (2) to identify students who are moderately to severely dependent on alcohol, who have been advised by a physician not to drink, or who present with health conditions (e.g., possible pregnancy, ulcers, diabetes) where any use of alcohol could be medically contraindicated.

Although feedback and advice are not technically provided until the second meeting, the clinical frame begins developing the moment the student walks into the room where the sessions are to be held and is greeted by the therapist. For this reason, it is important that the therapist attend to creating rapport as much as gaining information about the student through the specific interview procedures. Ensuring, for example, that the client feels safe to talk freely about his or her experiences and feels "heard" will pay off handsomely in the quality of data obtained. It is important to remember that whereas a therapist may perceive himself or herself as "open," "liberal," "non-judgmental," and so on, a student may come primed from past experiences to expect that the therapist has an unstated "agenda" or will ultimately advocate absolute abstinence, as the student has heard from other prevention messages.

The approach to this first session is consistent with that of typical structured clinical interviews. We like to think about these intake sessions as we might think of a road trip: We start out with a clear destination in mind, and follow the basic course we have charted on our map. However, we may choose to drive more slowly at certain points or to pull off the road entirely to take in a particular sight. We may also decide to take a slight detour or to go down a path we hadn't originally intended, because we see something interesting we want to take in more closely. In this sense, the interview and assessment measures, like the map, provide the basic structure. They should not, however, be used like a blueprint that is intended to be followed to a "T." Side trips, stopping, and slowing down to take particular note of something of clinical interest are all strongly encouraged.

Because many factors contribute to heavy and hazardous drinking among college students—from alcohol expectancies to a student's place of residence—it is important to listen carefully to the narrative presented by the student for information about the context in which drinking occurs. This should include information about how the student interacts with his or her environment, both when drinking and when not drinking. The therapist should seek to understand the student's world (including aspects of his or her life outside of drinking activities), and especially the factors that may result in heavy drinking and the barriers that may compromise efforts to moderate use.

As part of the task of understanding who the student is, the therapist should be listening for what we might think of as the student's "motivational incentives" to drink moderately. General incentives include, for example, spending less money on alcohol, getting better grades, and wanting to avoid humiliating social situations (e.g., vomiting in front of a prospective dating partner, etc.). The therapist need not address these incentives at this point, but instead should simply listen carefully for information that may be relevant during the subsequent session, when the therapist aims to increase the student's interest in reducing risky drinking. **Simply put, the therapist should be awake and alert during this first session, seeking clues to a motivational "hook" to use in making the case for change during the second session.**

How does the therapist go about eliciting this kind of information? Although the main purpose of the session is to collect information about the student's level of risk and pattern of consumption, opportunities occasionally arise to provide the student with some information about alcohol and/or its effects. We do not recommend that this become a dominant focus of this first session. Rather, if the opportunity presents itself, the therapist should not hesitate to take a few minutes to answer a student's questions about alcohol or to provide a piece of information, with assurances that more time can be spent on these issues during the second session. Information provided at this point should "fit" within the context of the assessment discussion, as opposed to creating opportunities to insert this information (as we intentionally do in the second meeting).

PREPARING FOR THE FIRST SESSION

Depending on the purpose for which the brief intervention is performed, the initial interview may focus specifically on drinking behaviors (e.g., typical drinking pattern and atypical or episodic drinking occasions), alcohol-related risks, and negative consequences occurring as a result of drinking alcohol. In other situations and for other purposes, this interview may cover a broader range of lifestyle behaviors (e.g., smoking, use of other substances, eating disorders, use of alcohol within the context of dating, etc.). In our own clinical work utilizing BASICS, we have tended to use a "bare-bones" approach. Our decision to limit the assessment in most cases to questions relating only to alcohol has been driven primarily by time and cost restrictions. When time and other resources allow, we incorporate a broader range of lifestyle behaviors into the initial assessment. We encourage users of this manual to direct the interview toward either their own projects' specific aims or their students' specific needs.

Because our main research interests involve reducing harmful effects from heavy drinking, we have naturally focused throughout the brief intervention on alcohol use. For the purposes of our Lifestyles research, the initial face-to-face interview with students included an assessment of the following:

- Typical drinking pattern, and atypical or episodic drinking occasions, for the past 30 days.

- Indices of alcohol dependence.

- History of conduct disorder.

- History of alcohol and/or mental health problems.

- Family history of alcohol or other substance use problems and/or mental health problems.

The initial self-report questionnaire packet completed by students participating in the Lifestyles Project following the face-to-face interview assessed the factors listed below. (Although this packet is optimally administered after the initial interview, once rapport is established, self-report measures can also be given to students before the interview begins.)

- Assorted drinking variables (frequency, quantity, etc.).

- Negative consequences resulting from alcohol use over the past 6 months.

- Use of other psychoactive substances in the past 6 months.

- Sexual behaviors, including risky sex behaviors involving alcohol and other drug use.

- Alcohol outcome expectancies.

- Perception of health and behavioral risks due to alcohol.

- Interest in changing, and degree of readiness to change, drinking.

- Perceptions of college drinking norms.

- Symptoms of psychological distress.

- Indices of alcohol dependence.

As is evident from the two lists, assessments of alcohol use and alcohol dependence were included in both the face-to-face interview and the self-report paper-and-pencil screening. Our original purpose for using overlapping measures was to increase the reliability of the data for research purposes. We have also found that the approaches complement each other. For example, the interview procedure used to assess the typical drinking pattern lends itself nicely to obtaining more precise data, as the interviewer can ensure that each student is using the same definition of **standard drink** in approximating his or her use. However, some students may feel uncomfortable openly acknowledging their heavy use to an interviewer, but may be willing to record their best guesses in the context of a "private" questionnaire.

THE ACTUAL MEETING

Rapport Building, Orienting, and Getting an Initial Commitment

In addition to gathering information about the student, three clinical goals for the first meeting are (1) building rapport with the student, (2) orienting the student to the purpose and structure of the meetings, and (3) gaining an initial commitment from the student to participate in the intervention. In regard to building rapport with a student, it is helpful to remember that many students have never previously met with a mental health or public health practitioner and may have a fair amount of uncertainty about what to expect. In some of our cases where students had received previous counseling, they described their experiences in somewhat negative terms, on account of "not knowing what to say or do" during the session. It is not uncommon for students to arrive to the initial meeting expecting to hear a "Just Say No" plea for abstinence, or a repetition of material covered in their high school health classes. Our students have occasionally commented, for example, "I've heard this stuff in high school. Why do I have to do this again?" Although this issue is of particular relevance during the second meeting, we believe it is imperative for the therapist to address this issue early, whether directly or indirectly, if it is on the student's mind. One strategy is to invite the student to identify what is "new" and "old" information.

In the spirit of building rapport and orienting students to our basic aim and interest in BASICS, we have found it helpful to state in some fashion at an early opportunity that our intention isn't to **make** them do anything. Instead, we underscore the following two points:

- Although we make strategies for safer drinking available to the each student, the student gets to decide whether he or she wants to change or even wants to consider changing.

- The decision about what to do with the information provided belongs entirely to the student.

We emphasize that students frequently learn to drink in haphazard ways, usually by experimenting on their own or by watching others. Whereas most students learn how to drive safely to prevent accidents and problems, few actually learn how to drink safely. We do not tell them, for example, what they should or shouldn't do, but instead seek to provide them with information on which to base their decisions.

In recent applications of BASICS, we have drawn from the work of Marsha Linehan (1993), a colleague of ours at the University of Washington, in emphasizing orienting and commitment strategies throughout the intervention. Although orienting and commitment are separate procedures, they typically occur hand in hand with each other. Orienting involves providing the student with the essential lay of the land, some sense of what to expect, and what is being asked of him or her, in order to maximize the likelihood that the student will be able to receive and make use of the brief intervention. Linehan (1993) has observed that "many apparent failures to learn stem from failures to understand what has to be learned, rather than problems with acquisition or memory" (p. 283). Before the student can be motivated to moderate use of alcohol, he or she first needs to understand something about the brief intervention procedure.

Obtaining an initial commitment from the student to collaborate in the intervention is the third therapist goal for the early portion of the first session. This commitment may include providing thoughtful answers during the initial interview, joining the therapist in the process of weighing the evidence about risks, and/or evaluating the pros and cons of considering changes in his or her drinking pattern. For students who wish to learn new behavioral strategies or skills, commitment can also include agreeing to work on learning and applying the new skills. Making a commitment to do something increases the probability that the behavior will actually be performed in the future (e.g., Wang & Katzev, 1990; Hall, Havassy, & Wasserman, 1990). Simply stated, people are more likely to do what they commit themselves to doing (Linehan, 1993). For this reason, it is important for students to have a real choice about whether they participate—and, if so, how they participate. In the case of students who are mandated to seek treatment, genuine commitment to participate is made difficult by the real constraints on choice; nevertheless, it is not impossible even in this situation and should be sought. At the most fundamental level, choices do exist—both whether to receive BASICS as a sanction (as opposed, say, to being expelled from a residence hall) and how fully to participate. Here are some of the strategies we use in such a case:[1]

Step 1. The therapist simply and playfully reminds the student that although the consequence (participating in treatment) is not very desirable, a choice does nonetheless exist; at the same time, the therapist empathizes with the constraints being imposed, which make the student question whether or not there really is a choice but to participate.

> THERAPIST: So you aren't really thrilled about doing this. You know you do have a choice. It's probably not the choice you wanted, but you do have one nonetheless. The reality is that you could find another place to live that you may like even better than this place.

> STUDENT: Yeah, I could, but that would be a big hassle. Then I'd have to tell my parents about this and everything else.

> THERAPIST: You could do that, but this is sort of the lesser of two evils, right? Makes sense to me.

> STUDENT: Yeah. This is a lot easier and a lot less hassle than moving out and dealing with my parents over this.

Step 2. The therapist then secures the student's agreement to make the most of the intervention.

> THERAPIST: You're right! This is definitely the easier path. A couple of hours and you're finished. I send a letter to your head resident, and that's that. Since that is the path you're selecting—even though you aren't nuts about it—I wonder if we could have an agreement that we will make the most of it.

> STUDENT: Yeah, I suppose. It's not like I'm going to sleep through it or something.

> THERAPIST: Well, I suppose you could if you wanted to. The issue is really this: Unlike students who come to see me because they want to, your circum-

---

[1]The first author wishes to acknowledge the significant contribution of Linehan's commitment strategies in *Dialectical Behavior Therapy* and her influence in our work in securing a behavioral commitment in BASICS. Readers who are interested in learning more about obtaining a commitment with difficult-to-treat populations are encouraged to read Linehan's (1993) discussion of these strategies in her treatment manual, *Cognitive-Behavioral Treatment of Borderline Personality Disorder.*

stances are different, just as we've discussed. What you get out of this depends largely on what you put into it. Although I too would prefer that you were wildly excited about being here, I accept that you're not, and I'm willing to work just as hard to be helpful. I'd like for you to do the same. So rather than assuming something of you, I'd like us to have an agreement to maximize this time together.

Step 3. The therapist finds out whether the student has any questions or curiosities that can be addressed during the brief intervention.

> THERAPIST: I wonder if you have any questions or topics related to alcohol use that are of particular interest to you. If you do, I want to make sure that you and I have a chance to address them.

As part of building commitment, efforts are made to elicit the student's cooperation in implementing the behavioral solutions discussed as part of the intervention. Put simply, the therapist seeks the student's agreement to try out a new behavior or to work on a specific problem, rather than assuming agreement. Because of the time-limited, minimal intervention nature of BASICS, there are limited opportunities to devise and test out specific behavioral solutions during the course of the student's work with the therapist. Therefore, the student is asked for a broader commitment to testing and then refining behavioral strategies until an approach is found that works well for him or her. This level of commitment is typically sought during the second meeting, when the student receives feedback and advice; the student agrees to try out specific modifications to the way in which he or she drinks.

A sample dialogue (Dialogue 4.1) illustrates the overall process of building rapport, orienting, and seeking commitment.

Dialogue 4.1. Building Rapport, Orienting, and Seeking Commitment

> THERAPIST: One important reason for our meeting is to talk together about risks associated with drinking, and about aspects of your drinking style that either have already resulted or may result in the future in unpleasant or harmful experiences for you. If you are interested, I'd like to think with you about ways to maybe minimize the likelihood of having unpleasant outcomes from drinking. In our experience, people often learn how to drink by experimenting or by watching others—sort of by trial and error, and unfortunately sometimes with a lot of error. What about you? How did you learn how to drink alcohol?

> STUDENT: I don't know. I guess I learned by hanging around a group of people who drank. I just watched them and did what they did.

> THERAPIST: That's pretty common. Most of the time, watching what others do is a

good way to learn something new. With alcohol, however, it doesn't always result in learning how to avoid unpleasant outcomes. Drinking can be like driving a really fun car. It's exciting and fun, but accidents and bad times can happen if people are having so much fun that they aren't also focused on safety. We like to give students who drink alcohol some basic training in how to do it safely, similar to what you may have received in driver's education back in high school. The goal, of course, is to focus on ways to drink that would allow you to enjoy the experience without having to encounter unwanted effects or harmful consequences from the alcohol. What do you think about that?

STUDENT: I'm not too worried about it. I learned some stuff about alcohol while I was in high school. They basically told us not to drink, or at least not to drink and drive. I'm basically covered, and I don't really need more information about what I should do. I never drink and drive because I live in the Greek system and can pretty much walk home from the parties I attend.

THERAPIST: That's great that you don't drink and drive. You know, many students find that what we focus on here is pretty different from what they got in high school. For example, I'm not going to tell you what you should or shouldn't do. What you do with the information we go over is really entirely up to you.

STUDENT: That's good. I hated those high school lectures and being told what to do.

THERAPIST: If you're open to it, my goal for the two of us would be to take a closer look at any ways in which your pattern of drinking results in good things and unpleasant or harmful experiences, and then to see if we might figure out some ways to increase the likelihood of the benefits and decrease the likelihood of these unwanted experiences from drinking. For me to be able to be of greatest assistance, it's important that I can get a much clearer sense of the tradeoffs of your drinking style and some additional information that we have found useful in thinking about students' risks. How does that sound?

STUDENT: I see what you're saying. That sounds fine, I guess.

Assessing High-Risk Lifestyle and Health Behaviors

As previously mentioned, the exact components of the assessment will naturally vary, given the scope and context of the intervention and the time available for conducting BASICS. The assessment measures reviewed in this manual are among those utilized in our research and clinical work. The measures were selected on the basis of their strong psychometric properties. A full list of possible measures for use is included in Appendix A; the review below focuses only on those measures that require a somewhat detailed interviewing process.

Assessment of Typical Drinking Pattern and Episodic Drinking Occasions

Various methods exist for assessing alcohol consumption, each with particular strengths and limitations (see NIAAA, 1995, for a review of this literature). Tradeoffs usually involve balancing the degree of specificity the researcher/clinician wishes to obtain against the time and resources available. The obvious question in deciding which route to take is simply this: "How do I want to make use of this information?" We recommend a method that sheds light on the way a student drinks, in addition to how much he or she consumes. We often use the typical and episodic drinking measures from the Brief Drinker Profile (BDP; Miller & Marlatt, 1984), each of which takes an average of 5–7 minutes to complete.

The first task is to use the Steady Pattern Chart portion of the BDP (see Figure 4.1) to map the student's typical pattern of drinking over the past 30 days, using standardized drink measurements (e.g., one **standard drink** is equivalent to 12 ounces of standard beer, 4 ounces of wine, 1¼ ounces of 80-proof alcohol, or 10 ounces of wine cooler). As displayed in Figure 4.1, the therapist records the type of beverage consumed (e.g., hard alcohol, beer, wine, etc.), the ounces consumed, and the time intervals when drinking typically occurs (e.g., from the time the person first typically takes a drink to the time he or she consumes the last drink in a particular drinking interval).

One way to use this portion of the BDP is to direct the student through a series of questions for each of the 21 intervals (3 intervals daily over 7 days) given for a typical week in Figure 4.1—starting with the upper left box, completing the day, then moving to the morning of the following day, and so on. Because college students typically drink alcohol in a fairly standard, predictable fashion (e.g., weekend nights, after finals, before big sporting events), it may be more efficient to begin by asking the student a general question about when he or she typically drinks, in order to get "the lay of the land." The therapist can then fill in the relevant cells, and can conclude by asking the student whether there are any other occasions when he or she typically drinks alcohol that have not yet been discussed.

As is always the case when beginning a new series of questions in the interview, we recommend orienting the student to the assessment task by offering a brief overview and rationale for the task. The explanation for the BDP should also include an operational definition for *standard drink* (as previously defined), **typical pattern,** and **episodic occasions,** to further ensure accuracy of data. By **typical pattern,** we mean using alcohol in a fairly consistent way more than half the time in the past 30 days. So if a student reported using alcohol in a reasonably consistent manner on three out of four Fridays in the past 30 days, we would record this as typical. However, if the student reported consuming the same amount on alternating Fridays, we would not record this as typical, but would instead record it as two occasions of episodic drinking (see Figure 4.2, below).

Brief Drinker Profile (Modified)

SUBJECT # ☐
GROUP # ☐
WEIGHT ☐

1. STEADY PATTERN CHART

If the client drinks at least once per week complete the Steady Pattern Chart, then complete Q/F data summary.
For each time period enter the type of beverage,
percentage of alcohol, amount consumed, and approximate time span during which it is consumed.

Time of Day	Sunday	Monday	Tuesday	Wednesday	Thursday	Friday	Saturday
Morning							
Afternoon							
Evening							
Daily SECs Totals							

FORMULA FOR CALCULATING SECs: Number of ounces multiplied by percentage of alcohol multiplied by 2 equals total number of SECs. (# oz. X % alcohol X 2 = SECs.)

A. Total SECs Per Week

Sunday
Monday
Tuesday
Wednesday
Thursday
Friday
Saturday
Total

A. TOTAL SECs per week . . . . ☐

B. TOTAL drinking (nonabstinent) days reported . . . . ☐

C. AVERAGE SECs per Drinking Day . . . . ☐
(A divided by B)

FIGURE 4.1. The Brief Drinker Profile (BDP), Steady Pattern Chart portion. Q/F, quantity/frequency; SEC, standard ethanol consumption. Adapted and reproduced by special permission of the Publisher, Psychological Assessment Resources, Inc., 16204 North Florida Avenue, Lutz, Florida 33549, from the *Comprehensive Drinker Profile*. Copyright 1984. Further reproduction is prohibited without permission of the Publisher (except for photocopy rights to purchasers). Reprinted in *Brief Alcohol Screening and Intervention for College Students (BASICS): A Harm Reduction Approach* by Linda A. Dimeff, John S. Baer, Daniel R. Kivlahan, and G. Alan Marlatt. Copyright 1999 by The Guilford Press. Permission to photocopy this figure is granted to purchasers of *BASICS* for personal use only (see copyright page for details).

We define an **episodic occasion** as any occasion that involves either (1) drinking any amount of alcohol during a nontypical period, or (2) drinking more than the typical amount usually consumed (as previously recorded under the typical pattern), during the past 30 days. Students often relate tidbits indicating their episodic use of alcohol when describing their typical pattern of alcohol use. Dialogue 4.2 illustrates walking a student through the first portion of the BDP (the Steady Pattern Chart—Figure 4.1).

Dialogue 4.2. Getting the Typical Pattern of Alcohol Use with the BDP

THERAPIST: Now I'd like to ask you a series of questions that will help me get an idea of how and when you use alcohol. I'm first going to ask you about your typical pattern of drinking. By "typical," I mean what has usually been the case for you, more often than not. I would like you to use the last 30 days as your frame of reference. It's often helpful to establish a time anchor. In this case, 30 days takes us back to around Halloween. Right?

STUDENT: Yeah.

THERAPIST: Anything else going on around that time that would help you remember your drinking in the past 30 days?

STUDENT: Definitely! Homecoming. We had a big weekend party. Hmm . . . oh, and a big test in my geography class.

THERAPIST: Okay, good. Let's keep both of those events in mind as we map out your typical pattern of use. After we do that, I'll ask you some additional questions about other occasions during the last 30 days when you may have consumed more than what's typical for you. Finally, on the days that you do drink, I'll ask you some additional questions about what and how much you drank. I will want to record how much you drink in terms of "standard drinks." By that I mean 12 ounces of beer, 4 ounces of wine, 1¼ ounces of 80-proof hard liquor, or 10 ounces of wine coolers or beer. Okay, any questions so far?

STUDENT: No. Seems pretty clear so far.

THERAPIST: Okay, good. Thinking back over the last 30 days as your reference, what days do you typically drink on?

STUDENT: Mostly Friday and Saturday nights. Sometimes Wednesdays, but it sort of depends on what else is going on.

THERAPIST: Okay, let's start with Friday. How many drinks do you typically have on Friday?

STUDENT: About 8 beers.

THERAPIST: Are those standard 12-ounce cans of beer?

STUDENT: Yes.

THERAPIST: From when to when do you typically drink the beers on Friday?

STUDENT: Let's see. Probably from about 9:00 P.M. until about 1:00 A.M.

THERAPIST: Okay, so about 4 hours. Does that sound about right?

STUDENT: Yeah.

THERAPIST: Okay, what about Saturday?

STUDENT: The same for Saturday. Well, maybe one to two beers more.

THERAPIST: About 10 beers over the same period of 4 hours, from 9:00 P.M. until 1:00 A.M.?

STUDENT: Yeah, that's about right.

THERAPIST: You mentioned that you sometimes drink on Wednesdays. Thinking over the last 30 days, did you drink more often than not on Wednesdays?

STUDENT: Actually, no. I think only twice.

THERAPIST: Okay, so we won't record it now, but we'll come back to it later on. Now are there any other occasions during the last 30 days when you typically consumed alcohol that we haven't already talked about?

STUDENT: No, that's it.

THERAPIST: All right.

Once the typical pattern is obtained, the therapist then turns his or her attention to all other drinking occasions that did not fit the typical pattern during the same 30-day period—in other words, when the student had more to drink than the typical amount. To orient the student to the segue from the typical pattern to the episodic occasions, the therapist might state the following:

"Now that we've reviewed your typical pattern of drinking over the past 30 days, I want to go back and record all the occasions when you had more to drink than the typical pattern. This can include times when you drank more than your typical amount on a particular drinking day, or occasions when you drank that are not a part of your typical pattern."

Using the portion of the BDP illustrated in Figure 4.2, the therapist records information about the circumstances of each event (e.g., "It was the playoff game and we had a party for the whole hall"), as well as information about what types of drinks and how much alcohol were consumed over how many hours. Dialogue 4.3 illustrates walking a student through this portion of the BDP.

Episodic Pattern Chart

(Periodic and Combination Pattern Drinking)

SUBJECT #

GROUP #

2. QUANTITY/FREQUENCY OF EPISODIC DRINKING
Multiply Quantity (SECs per episode) by Frequency (episodes per 3 months) for each episode type.

SECs is the number of ounces multiplied by percentage of alcohol multiplied by two (# oz. X % alcohol X 2).
BAC is the blood/alcohol concentration. (Weight/sex/SECs/hours).

1. EPISODE TYPE ONE:

Brief description of episode:	
Type of beverage consumed:	Amount of time in episode **(hours)**:
Number of drinks consumed:	Number of SECs per drink	Total number SECs consumed per episode:
		Peak BAC during episode:
	Number of times in past 3 months this type of episode occurs:

2. EPISODE TYPE TWO:

Brief description of episode:	
Type of beverage consumed:	Amount of time in episode **(hours)**:
Number of drinks consumed:	Number of SECs per drink	Total number SECs consumed per episode:
		Peak BAC during episode:
	Number of times in past 3 months this type of episode occurs:

3. EPISODE TYPE THREE:

Brief description of episode:	
Type of beverage consumed:	Amount of time in episode **(hours)**:
Number of drinks consumed:	Number of SECs per drink	Total number SECs consumed per episode:
		Peak BAC during episode:
	Number of times in past 3 months this type of episode occurs:

FIGURE 4.2. The Brief Drinker Profile (BDP), portion. From Miller and Rollnick (1984). Adapted and reproduced by special permission of the Publisher, Psychological Assessment Resources, Inc., 16204 North Florida Avenue, Lutz, Florida 33549, from the *Comprehensive Drinker Profile*. Copyright 1984. Further reproduction is prohibited without permission of the Publisher (except for photocopy rights to purchasers). Reprinted in *Brief Alcohol Screening and Intervention for College Students (BASICS): A Harm Reduction Approach* by Linda A. Dimeff, John S. Baer, Daniel R. Kivlahan, and G. Alan Marlatt. Copyright 1999 by The Guilford Press. Permission to photocopy this figure is granted to purchasers of *BASICS* for personal use only (see copyright page for details).

Dialogue 4.3. Assessing Episodic Drinking Occasions with the BDP

THERAPIST: Now that we have recorded your typical pattern in the past 90 days, I want to go back over the 90-day period and record occasions when you had more to drink than the typical pattern. This can include times when you drank more than the typical amount on a typical drinking day, or other times when you drank when it wasn't one of your regular drinking days.

STUDENT: Let's see. I had a party in my room two Fridays ago for my friend who turned 21. It was pretty wild. I think I had between 12 and 15 beers that night.

THERAPIST: Do you think it was closer to 12 or 15?

STUDENT: Probably 15.

THERAPIST: Okay. Were you again drinking standard 12-ounce cans of beer?

STUDENT: Yes.

THERAPIST: Over what period of time were you drinking?

STUDENT: From about 9:00 P.M. until 2:30 A.M.

THERAPIST: Any other occasions during the past 90 days when you had more to drink than the typical pattern?

STUDENT: No, I don't think so.

Assessment of Alcohol Dependence

Although it is important to assess alcohol dependence, assessing it in college students is by no means simple. Younger adults may meet the official DSM-IV criteria for this disorder, but not the "spirit" or "intent" of this diagnostic category. Instead, young people's endorsement of items on measures of alcohol dependence is often somewhat idiosyncratic, and for this reason it requires closer scrutiny when an attempt at an accurate diagnosis is being made. Listed below are several excerpts from clinical interviews in which we have used questions from the Patient Edition of the Structured Clinical Interview for DSM-IV Axis I Disorders (SCID; First, Spitzer, Gibbon, & Williams, 1995) concerning alcohol dependence:

- *Have you ever found that when you started drinking, you ended up drinking much more than you were planning to?*

  I hardly ever think about how much I'm going to drink in advance. It just sort of depends on what's going on at the party and how much money we can pool together in advance to buy the alcohol.

- *Have you ever spent a lot of time drinking, being high, or hung over?*

  What do you mean by "a lot of time"? Usually during homecoming week, my fraternity hosts a lot of activities with our sister sorority. We usually start drinking midweek and keep drinking through the weekend!

- *Have you ever drunk so often that you drank instead of working or spending time at hobbies or with your family or friends?*

  I often miss my 8:00 A.M. class (because of a hangover), but I usually get the notes from someone else who went the days I miss.

- *Have you ever found that you needed to drink a lot more in order to get high, compared to when you first started drinking?*

  Compared to when I first started drinking? Well, yeah, of course. It used to take just a drink or two. Now it takes me about four just to start feeling it.

When a student does meet DSM-IV criteria for alcohol dependence, according to a self-report measure or a standardized interview procedure such as the SCID, we recommend that attention be paid to determining whether the student does indeed fit the "spirit" of this disorder (i.e., physical and/or psychological dependence).

Family History of Alcohol/Other Substance Use Problems and/or Psychopathology

The primary objective in assessing the student's family history of alcohol problems, other substance use problems, or mental health problems is to identify any biological and social influences that may place the student at additional risk for alcohol problems. For purposes of our research, we used the well-described Family Tree Questionnaire developed by Mann, Sobell, Sobell, and Pavan (1985). Briefly, this questionnaire obtains current and historical information on biological relatives with respect to their use of alcohol, their use of other substances, and their history of psychopathology. For each relative identified as having either alcohol or substance use problems, or a history of psychological difficulties, a separate and more detailed series of questions further clarifies the specific nature of that person's problems.

After orienting a student to the task of inquiring about family history of substance misuse and/or psychological difficulties, we then provide the student with some working definitions for what we mean by these terms. We have found this helpful in enhancing the quality of the information students provide about their families, in light of the varied understandings of these terms. Definitions we commonly give in our own clinical work are illustrated in Dialogue 4.4 (see below). It is also helpful to provide the student with a framework for **family** (e.g., adoptive, biological, etc.).

Once operational definitions are provided, the task then shifts to collecting the relevant history about the student's family members. Information can be gathered quickly and efficiently by clustering family members into groups (e.g., all grandparents, parents, aunts and uncles, and finally siblings), regardless (at first) of which side of the family

• • •

they are on. A general question can be asked for each of the groups that covers substance use and mental health problems (e.g., "Have any of them ever had difficulties with alcohol or other substances, or have any of your grandparents ever experienced psychological difficulties that compromised some aspect of their life functioning?"). Unless the student identifies a grandparent who did have one or more of these problems, the interviewer can then ask the same question about the parents, followed by aunts and uncles, and finally by siblings. Whenever a family member is identified as having one of the three specified difficulties, the interviewer can then pause to inquire more about the nature of the difficulties and about whether (if at all) the student personally experienced or was affected by these.

How much information should one gather from the student about the nature of a relative's problems? It is not necessary that the therapist know all there is to know about the relative's problems, or be able to assign a diagnosis. Instead, the clinician should ask enough questions to learn generally whether or not the relative indeed had a problem, and to what extent the problem(s) affected the relative's and the student's lives. One simple way to determine whether enough information has been gathered is to remember the primary clinical aim in gathering this information to begin with: to develop a motivational "hook" for use during the second session, which will increase the student's interest in changing his or her drinking pattern.

On occasion, a student will express a keen interest in talking about a particular relative's problem(s) and the ways in which the student's life was affected. In the interest of time and purpose of BASICS, we discourage therapists from asking questions of students that encourage "catharsis" or reexperiencing "what it was like." At the same time, we do encourage therapists to recognize and respect that for some students, a discussion of family history of behavioral and emotional difficulties may bring up unpleasant and perhaps painful feelings. In such a case, we recommend that the therapist take a moment to listen to the student, while refraining from "deepening" the discussion by avoiding additional questions or comments that require the student to express or reveal more. In such cases, it is likely that this content will be of considerable use as a motivational "hook" in the coming session.

Dialogue 4.4 illustrates the process of assessing a student's family history of alcohol/other substance use problems and/or psychopathology.

Dialogue 4.4. Assessing Family History of Alcohol/Other Substance Use Problems and/or Difficulties in Psychological Functioning

THERAPIST: Now I'd like to ask you some questions about your biological family and whether anyone in your family has ever experienced difficulties with alcohol or other drugs, or if anyone has ever had a history of psychological difficulties. When I say "family," I'm referring to all your blood relatives. Make sense?

STUDENT: I think so.

THERAPIST: Okay, good. Now different people often mean very different things by alcohol and drug problems. For our purposes here, I'm defining "problems" as behaviors that are causing difficulties in living for the person, or somehow compromises the person's ability to function as fully as he or she might otherwise be capable of doing. This might include family or marital difficulties, problems at work, legal problems, and so forth. So, as we're defining it, alcohol problems could include such things as divorce if the person's drinking was the reason for the divorce. Psychological problems could include missing work for an extended period due to depression. Any questions yet?

STUDENT: Nope. I'm still clear.

THERAPIST: Okay. A few points and we're ready to start. First, by "drugs," I'm including all drugs here, whether illegal or prescription. Finally, if you have any questions as we go along, do not hesitate to ask me. If you aren't sure, we can always stop and sort out something. Okay?

STUDENT: Okay.

THERAPIST: All right, then. Let's start with your grandparents. Have any of your grandparents ever had difficulties or problems with alcohol or other drugs, or psychological problems that you are aware of?

STUDENT: Hmm. My mom told me that her father was an alcoholic. She always told me to be careful so I wouldn't end up like him.

THERAPIST: So your maternal grandfather?

STUDENT: Right.

THERAPIST: What was problematic about his use of alcohol? Do you know?

STUDENT: I actually never met him. He died before I was born.

THERAPIST: Did you ever get a sense from your mother about what it was about his use of alcohol that made her suspect he had a problem?

STUDENT: She says he drank all the time and got wasted pretty often. She says sometimes he got pretty mean to my grandmother when he drank.

THERAPIST: Ah. I see. How about your other grandparents?

STUDENT: Nope. No problems with the rest. Just my mom's dad.

THERAPIST: What about your parents? Have your parents ever had difficulties with psychological problems, or difficulties with alcohol or drugs?

STUDENT: No. My mother didn't drink because she was afraid of being like her father.

THERAPIST: Okay. What about your aunts or uncles?

STUDENT: Not that I'm aware of.

THERAPIST: Now I can't tell if you don't know them well enough to know, or do know them but have no reason to believe any of them have had these difficulties.

STUDENT: I know them, but I haven't ever heard or seen anything to suggest any of them have these problems.

THERAPIST: Okay. And, finally, what about your siblings?

STUDENT: Well, my brother was seeing a psychologist for a while. I'm not sure for what. I think it had something to do with anxiety attacks, or something. He'd get really freaked out every time he took tests.

THERAPIST: Did the anxiety attacks hold him back or significantly get in his way, or was it more that he felt really uncomfortable but was able to work it though with the help of his doctor?

STUDENT: It wasn't really that big of a deal. I think he went for 3 or 4 months, or something. But he always did really well in school, even during the time that he had the attacks.

THERAPIST: I'm glad to hear it. Now have we missed anyone?

STUDENT: No. I think we touched on them all.

Monitoring Cards

Once the gathering of information about the student's own alcohol use and his or her family history is completed, the therapist requests that the student monitor his or her drinking on a daily basis from the close of the initial session up until the time of the subsequent meeting. The student is provided with approximately 20 wallet-sized monitoring cards, along with basic instructions in how to use the cards. As illustrated in Figure 4.3, each monitoring card contains columns for numerous situational factors that facilitate documenting the specific context in which the student's drinking occurs. Students are instructed to make at least an entry per day, indicating "none" for nondrinking days and completing a full row of responses per drinking occasion, indicating what they drank, where they were, who they were with, and what their mood was while drinking the beverage. Codes for common responses across these situations are provided on the back of the monitoring card for ease of recording.

The purpose of having students monitor their drinking is twofold. First, the simple task of recording a behavior increases self-awareness, which can in and of itself be sufficient to change the behavior. The term **reactivity** (Watson & Tharp, 1993; Mace &

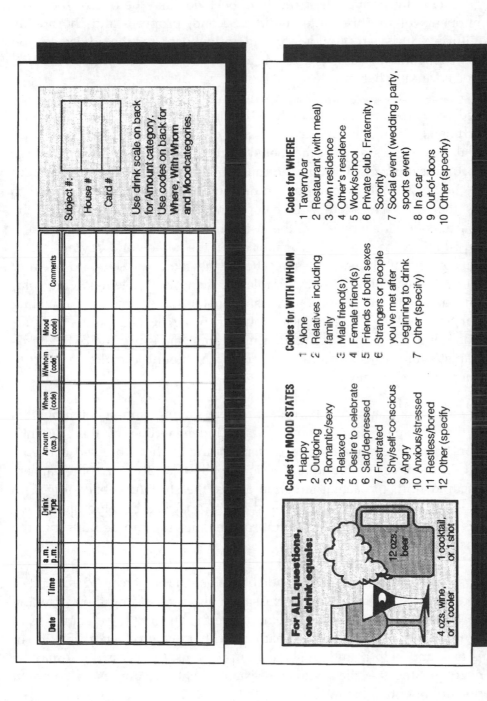

FIGURE 4.3. Both sides of monitoring cards for recording drinking behavior. From *Brief Alcohol Screening and Intervention for College Students (BASICS): A Harm Reduction Approach* by Linda A. Dimeff, John S. Baer, Daniel R. Kivlahan, and G. Alan Marlatt. Copyright 1999 by The Guilford Press. Permission to photocopy this figure is granted to purchasers of *BASICS* for personal use only (see copyright page for details).

Kratochwill, 1985) refers specifically to a decrease in unwanted behaviors and/or an increase in desired behaviors as a result of observing and recording them. For this reason, asking students to monitor their drinking behavior may be one of the more important components of the brief intervention. Second, properly and thoroughly completed monitoring cards can provide a useful springboard for the advice session by providing an avenue into discussing drinking and by furnishing additional context-specific data about drinking habits.

To a large degree, the cards are only meaningful to the extent that students make use of them. Unfortunately, students can tend to put off completing the cards until moments before the second session. In other behavior therapies, the therapist may have additional opportunities to work with a client on homework compliance; in BASICS, by contrast, the therapist has only one opportunity to "pitch" the homework and to address barriers that might interfere with completing the assignment. We use the following approach: Following a review of the instructions and rationale for self-monitoring, the therapist elicits the student's reactions about the homework. Paying careful attention to the content of the student's reactions, the therapist seeks to identify possible obstacles that may interfere with completing the task. Problem-solving solutions to these barriers are then discussed. In cases where the student remains unwilling to monitor his or her drinking, the therapist should then seek to negotiate a compromise between not monitoring at all and monitoring in an ideal fashion. Once the terms are set, the therapist again seeks a commitment from the student to make an effort to monitor his or her drinking behavior.

Throughout the process of identifying barriers, problem solving, and negotiating, it is important that the therapist clearly communicate understanding of the student's concerns. We aim to balance empathy and understanding of the expressed concerns with a sense that solutions can be found and seriously pursued. Because some barriers will remain obscured until the actual situation arises, the student is encouraged to experiment and solve problems as best he or she can *in vivo* to develop alternative solutions. Efforts to tinker with the plan to improve monitoring can be built into the commitment made by the student.

Common barriers described by students include objections to the perceived amount of time required to complete the task or embarrassment about recording their drinking while in public. Although it is important to emphasize the benefits to be gained from this exercise, a therapist must always empathize with the perceived difficulty of completing this task and help a student solve any problems. On occasion, it may be necessary to negotiate the specifics with a resistant client. Responses to common student concerns are described below.

- *How much time will this take?*

  We find that it only takes a minute or two to complete the information for each day you drink. As you familiarize yourself with the codes, it will probably take you even less time.

• *I'd feel a little strange recording drinking in front of everyone. Can't I do it the following day?*

It may be kind of embarrassing to do this publicly. Is that right?

• *Well, yeah.*

You could do it the next day. You may not get as much out of the exercise by doing it that way. That's my biggest concern. I wonder if there might be a way that you could keep track in a way that wouldn't result in embarrassment.

• *Well, I suppose I could dodge into the bathroom occasionally during a party and write down what I've had to drink. That might work.*

That sounds like a fine solution!

In Dialogue 4.5, the therapist validates the student's concerns and apprehensions about monitoring, and looks for an alternative that would be acceptable to both the student and the therapist. The therapist assumes a stance of "Let's put our heads together"—that is, working collaboratively with the student in the construction of a plan. Recognizing that the student may feel pressured or compelled to accept a plan prematurely, the therapist provides another opportunity to modify the plan, or for the student to express additional concerns. Finally, the therapist seeks a commitment from the student both to do the homework and to call the therapist if problems arise. The commitment is made "softly" (e.g., "Can we agree to that?") rather than forcefully, in an effort to minimize psychological reactance.

Dialogue 4.5. Self-Monitoring: Describing the Task and Getting a Commitment

THERAPIST: Okay, we're just about done for today. I have one more topic to talk with you about. I would like to request that you monitor and record your drinking between now and the time we meet again. There really are several reasons why it helps to do this. First and most importantly, it will help us both to get a better idea of how you drink. This information will be useful for us to look at when we meet the next time. In addition, people learn a lot about themselves when they actually take note of a particular behavior in this way. You may learn some things that you didn't already know, or may clarify some things that you have already considered. What were your thoughts about this as I was presenting you with this request?

STUDENT: I don't know. I don't know if I had any specific thoughts. What's involved?

THERAPIST: Good question. Basically, I'd like you to use these cards (*the therapist displays the monitoring cards*) to record your drinking. Essentially the task is to complete a row for each drink you have, recording here the date and time, the type and amount of alcohol you consumed, where you were, who you were with, and how you were feeling. To make this easier, we have listed a number of descriptions with codes here on the back (*the therapist displays the codes*) to make it a lot easier to record. On days when you don't drink, you'll just indicate the date and note "didn't drink." Other questions or thoughts before we continue?

STUDENT: Not about filling it out. That seems pretty straightforward.

THERAPIST: Okay, good. Now, ideally, it is usually best if you can actually do the recording as close as possible to the time that you actually have the drink.

STUDENT: You mean pull out the card and fill it out while I'm partying?

THERAPIST: Ideally, yes. What do you think about that? Does that seem like something you would be able to do?

STUDENT: Well, it might be a little awkward. I'm not sure I really want to do it right there. Is there some other way to do this?

THERAPIST: Yes, sure. What I just described is the ideal circumstance in terms of accuracy. The more time that lapses from the time you had the actual drink to the time you record it, the more it becomes difficult to remember exactly what you felt, when you had the drink, etc. However, what I also hear you saying is that this could compromise how much fun you might have, or that you might feel kind of awkward. I definitely want to figure out a way for you to do this that doesn't result in you having a bad experience. If that happens, then the whole point of the assignment becomes moot and not very helpful. Now, let's see. There are at least two possible issues. The first is compromising your fun by having to interrupt the moment and sort of disengage from the activity to do the recording. The second is how you'd feel—kind of awkward, completing the cards in front of your friends. Is that a fair summary?

STUDENT: That's pretty much it. I really think it's more the first one. I don't really care what my friends would think. They'd probably say something about it, like, "Hey, what's that?" I could tell them; they wouldn't really care. But I don't really want to stop what I'm doing to write down what I'm doing. You know what I mean?

THERAPIST: Yes, I think so. It sounds like you're okay with recording your drinks in general, but just not at the time that you're drinking. Is that right?

STUDENT: Yeah, that's pretty much it.

THERAPIST: Okay, so then we need to figure out a way for you not to have to sort of "leave" the party mentally or disengage in order to do this. At the same time, we need to think about how you can "collect the data," so to speak, in a way that makes it as accurate as possible. What do you think? Any suggestions about how you might accomplish both?

STUDENT: I don't know. Ah . . . maybe I could do it the following morning. I'll still pretty much remember what was going on.

THERAPIST: That's certainly one way to do it. My only concern with that plan is that things often look kind of different the following morning when a person's sober. What people remember of the experience is oftentimes really different from what they were experiencing at the time. Another possibility would be to only record your drinks one time during the party, and again the following morning. So you might, for example, decide to find a private, quiet place two-thirds of the way into the party and record everything up to that point. You could finish up the recording the following morning for the remaining one-third. That way, you could sizably minimize the disrupting aspect, but be closer to the actual event to reflect on the questions. How does that seem?

STUDENT: Yeah, that makes sense. I could go to the bathroom or someplace, and complete them there. Yeah, I think I could do that.

THERAPIST: Okay, good, then. Now does this seem like something you could commit to doing between now and the next time we meet? If there is something that still doesn't sit right with you, we can give some more thought now to how we might make it more workable for you.

STUDENT: No, I think this will work. Yeah, I can commit to doing it.

THERAPIST: Great. Okay, one final word about monitoring. You might find that once you actually put this to the test, you discover it doesn't work as well as we thought it might. I really want to encourage you to keep experimenting with improving the plan until it does fit. You might have to get even more creative. If you find that you're kind of stuck, I want you to call me so we can put our heads together and come up with something that might work better. Can we agree to that as well?

STUDENT: Yeah, but I don't think it will be a problem.

THERAPIST: Right. I think this plan we've worked out seems really reasonable, and you seem pretty clear about where the difficulties might emerge. I too have confidence in the plan. I also want to make sure we've got a backup plan in the event that we haven't considered something.

STUDENT: Oh, I see.

Wrapping Up the Initial Interview

Before bringing the opening interview to a close, the therapist should make arrangements for the second appointment. In order to obtain a good sampling of drinking behavior for monitoring, we recommend that the second session be scheduled no sooner than 10 days after the first interview. We prefer allowing 2 weeks between sessions so that the monitoring can include two weekends, since weekend days are

• • •

typically the days of heaviest drinking for college students. We also recommend that the therapist provide an additional opening for the student to express any concerns or questions he or she has up to that point. The therapist might close by stating the following:

> "We finally come to the ending of our first meeting. I enjoyed meeting you and appreciated your openness here with me. We've covered a lot of ground today. Before I get you started on completing some additional questionnaires, I want to check in with you and find out from you whether you have any questions or thoughts about anything we talked about or didn't get a chance yet to discuss."

By providing this invitation to speak freely about the process and content of the session, and to introduce other topics, the therapist creates another opportunity both to build rapport with the student and to obtain any additional information about the student that may be important in the final feedback and advice session.

SELF-REPORT QUESTIONNAIRE PACKET OF LIFESTYLE MEASURES

We recommend that a quiet, private room or area be made available to the student as he or she completes additional paper-and-pencil self-report measures. The questionnaire packet used in our research (see Table 4.1) was fairly comprehensive and took approximately 45 minutes to complete. Although this was necessary for research purposes, it is reasonable to produce a packet that requires less time to complete. As always, the decision of what to include in the packet should be guided by the primary aims of the intervention and the resources available. Again, all of our assessment measures are reviewed in Appendix A, along with a brief rationale for including the measures we used in our research.

STUDENT FEEDBACK ABOUT THE ASSESSMENT PROCEDURES

Whenever we conduct research studies with college students, we also attempt to learn how participants view the project and suggestions they recommend for future studies. In our Lifestyles research on BASICS, approximately 15 students provided feedback about their impressions of the assessment procedure. Several of the more frequently made comments are described below. It is important to remember that these comments were made by research participants who completed numerous measures. Because research participants are asked to complete more extensive assessment measures than students receiving BASICS for preventive or clinical purposes, the comments regarding assessment should be considered in this light.

1. *"The questionnaire packet gave me the feeling that you guys thought we had a big problem."* Many students indicated that the overemphasis on "pathological" or problematic behaviors in the assessment packet conveyed a message that we assumed they

TABLE 4.1. Summary of Self-Administered Measures Used in BASICS Research

Measure	Variable(s) assessed	Description	Estimated time required	Comments
Daily Drinking Questionnaire (Collins, Parks, & Marlatt, 1985)	Drinking variables (frequency, quantity, etc.)	Student indicates typical pattern of alcohol use for each day of the week in the past 30 days.	3 minutes	Has been modified to include typical hours spent drinking alcohol on each day indicated, to achieve estimate of BAL.
Frequency–Quantity Questionnaire (Cahalan & Cisin, 1968)	Drinking variables	Respondent endorses typical frequency and quantity of use in a specified period of time (e.g., typical month, typical weekend).	2 minutes	Considered quite a reliable and efficient means of gathering information about crude pattern of use.
Rutgers Alcohol Problems Inventory (White & Labouvie, 1989)	Common problems students experience when drinking	A 23-item measure developed specifically for student drinkers to assess more usual problems from alcohol. Includes assessment of alcohol dependence, concern about drinking, irresponsibility and/or neglect, and interpersonal conflict.	5 minutes	Excellent measure for research and clinical purposes. Because it was developed for young people, items are more relevant to their lifestyle than items in many other measures of problems.
Alcohol Dependence Scale (Skinner & Horn, 1984)	Alcohol dependence	A 25-item measure aimed at a variety of behaviors and experiences associated with alcohol dependence. Respondents are asked to endorse one of several answers that best represents their experience.	5 minutes	Widely used measure with strong psychometric properties. Whereas many of the questions ask about recent experiences, several provide no specific time parameters.
Readiness to Change Questionnaire (Rollnick, Heather, Gold, & Hall, 1992)	Motivation to change drinking habits	A 12-item measure based on Prochaska and DiClemente's stages of change	3 minutes	Important information for a clinician before meeting with a student; enables clinician to determine quickly where to focus clinical intervention, so as to gain greatest mileage from intervention.

(continued)

TABLE 4.1. *continued*

Measure	Variable(s) assessed	Description	Estimated time required	Comments
Drinking Norms Rating Form (Baer, Stacy, & Larimer, 1991)	Student perception of normative alcohol use by other college students	A 10-item measure assessing student's perception of typical drinking habits (e.g., frequency and quantity) for students of the same sex across a variety of dimensions (e.g., college-bound senior in high school, member of a fraternity/sorority, average student living in a dorm, respondent's closest friends, etc.). Student also specifies where he or she currently resides.	5 minutes	Excellent source of feedback to student, particularly when respondent endorses higher levels of use than actual normative levels among college students.
Comprehensive Effects from Alcohol (Fromme, Stroot, & Kaplan, 1993)	Alcohol outcome expectancies	A 38-item measure that spans eight different positive and negative alcohol outcome expectancies.	10 minutes	Although a sound and comprehensive measure, too lengthy for brief interventions. May be more useful for research purposes or as part of extensive clinical evaluations.
Alcohol Perceived Risks Problems (Duthie, Baer, & Marlatt, 1991)	Student self-appraisal of risk for developing alcohol problems	A 16-item measure asking students to rate the likelihood that they will experience specific problems from drinking alcohol while at college.	4 minutes	Provides professional with glimpse into student's own awareness of risks for problems from heavy drinking.
Brief Symptoms Inventory (Derogatis & Spencer, 1982)	Psychological distress	A 49-item measure covering eight clinical domains, including depression, anxiety, hostility, somatization. Includes several normed indices.	8 minutes	Excellent measure to assess self-reported global and specific symptoms of psychological distress. May be too lengthy for clinical brief interventions only. May consider use of specific subscales for more common problems, such as depression and anxiety.

were troubled. Ironically, we went to considerable lengths **not** to emphasize problems; we chose to talk about risks (and strategies to reduce risks) rather than assigning labels. Furthermore, we deliberately embedded the assessment of drinking behavior and negative consequences in a context of lifestyle behaviors. Students who raised this concern suggested that we also include "positive" items that would allow them to tell us "things we're doing right." One student suggested that the assessment could have included a measure of responsible drinking.

2. *"The questionnaire packet was too repetitive."* A number of students questioned why we asked the same questions twice. Was it because we didn't believe them? Were we trying to trick them? Or was it to make sure they paid attention and kept on their toes? Of course, the truth is that we did not ask the same exact questions twice. We did, however, ask the same **sorts** of questions several different ways. Although we did this for the sake of the research (to maintain the psychometric properties of each instrument we were using), it was nevertheless annoying to some of our participants. When we explained the rationale for the repetition, some students recommended that we simply acknowledge up front that the questionnaire packet is repetitive and provide an explanation, in words to this effect:

> "Each page of this packet contains a separate measure. We recognize that some of the questions may seem like 'repeats.' In order to preserve the integrity of each measure, we need to include the full measure, just as it was originally developed. We appreciate your patience in advance."

3. *"Your questions didn't really give me a chance to explain what I meant!"* Some students expressed frustration that the questions we asked were too narrow in focus and did not allow for a more complex understanding of the behavior in question. One student indicated, for example, that "the survey didn't ask me about the types of situations I drink in." Provision of open-ended responses for students to complete in order to "explain" their responses would easily address this concern.

CHAPTER 5

The Feedback Interview

We now turn our attention to the second session, where the therapist provides the student with feedback and advice about his or her drinking as assessed in the previous meeting. Following a review of the objectives and an overview of this meeting, we then focus on the therapist's preparation for this session. The third section reviews the workings of the actual meeting, from the content to examples of how to phrase particular portions of feedback.

Objectives and Overview of the Second Session

Preparing for the Second Session
Reviewing Assessment Materials and Generating Hypotheses
Guidelines for Selection of Drinking Goals
Using Computer-Generated Graphic Feedback
Developing a Personalized Blood Alcohol Level Chart and Card
Providing a "Tips" Sheet

The Actual Meeting
Orienting, Reestablishing Rapport, and Strengthening Commitment
Clinical Process and Approach to Providing Feedback and Advice
Providing Feedback and Advice
Making Referrals
Taking the Next Step: Stepped Care

OBJECTIVES AND OVERVIEW OF THE SECOND SESSION

We have named the second session of BASICS the **feedback session** to capture one of the primary aims of this meeting. We attempt to meet four objectives within this session:

1. Providing students with personalized feedback about their pattern of alcohol use and the risks associated with use. This includes comparing the quantity and frequency of the student's use to those of a normative sample of college

students, in addition to reviewing individual risk factors (e.g., positive alcohol outcome expectancies, family history of alcohol problems, personal history of negative or undesirable consequences of drinking, etc.).

2. Debunking myths and increasing the student's base of accurate information about alcohol and its effects.

3. Offering specific strategies to reduce current and future risks related to alcohol use.

4. Increasing the student's motivation to change current risky behaviors, and problem solving about potential barriers that might compromise initiation or maintenance of change.

The feedback session is idiographic; in other words, it is tailored to the student's particular needs. Therapists frequently weave feedback and advice-giving together throughout the second meeting, blending a touch of feedback with a dash of advice. Generally, more feedback is provided during the first portion of the interview. Advice-giving and making plans beyond BASICS are emphasized toward the end of the interview. Information about alcohol and its effects, motivational interviewing techniques, and barrier-removing strategies are embedded throughout the session. Although this chapter should serve as a basic guide to the interview, therapists are again encouraged to depart from the structure suggested here as they see fit, in order to respond to students' individual characteristics or needs.

In many regards, this second session is comparable to a patient's receiving feedback from a health care provider about a particular health concern, such as hypertension. In this scenario, the health care provider is likely first to notify the patient that his or her blood pressure is unusually high, and then to explain the specific medical risks posed by this condition. The provider may review factors that may account for the current condition (e.g., family history of hypertension, current fast-paced lifestyle, improper diet, etc.). Once this feedback is provided, the provider may identify a range of intervention options of increasing invasiveness (e.g., reduced salt intake, modest weight loss, very restrictive diets, antihypertensive medications, surgery); then discuss and negotiate an appropriate course of action to take to lower the blood pressure; and, finally, then continue to monitor and track the client's progress. Miller's Brief Drinker's Check-Up follows this general pattern (see Sobell & Sobell, 1993; Miller, Sovereign, & Krege, 1988).

PREPARING FOR THE SECOND SESSION

Reviewing Assessment Materials and Generating Hypotheses

In addition to the review of alcohol consumption habits and risks, the therapist should also thoroughly review all other information gathered from the student that will assist in forming additional impressions about him or her, or deepen the therapist's understanding of the role alcohol plays in the student's life or the context in which heavy drinking occurs. Sometimes in our work with high-risk drinkers, we find that students have apparently scaled back their drinking prior to our first meeting. On the surface of things, it would appear that these students have "matured" through the window of risk and are at relatively low risk. A review of the "secondary" questionnaires, however, may reveal information that might lead us to suspect that the light drinking is related not to an enduring pattern of change, but instead to temporary factors. This is a particularly common finding among student athletes, who typically abstain during competitive seasons.

Guidelines for Selection of Drinking Goals

The goal of moderation training is nonabusive, nonproblematic drinking. Obviously, not all students with alcohol problems are capable of moderating their use, despite their desire to do so. As a rule, college students who drink are not interested in abstaining from alcohol and prefer moderation, given a choice between the two. The key issue is determining when to recommend abstinence. The guidelines below represent the criteria we use in deciding when to advise abstinence; when therapists are in doubt, we encourage them to consult with a colleague or a physician, especially in cases where medical conditions complicate the picture.

- A student is experiencing moderate to severe alcohol dependence.

- A female student is pregnant or has reason to believe she is pregnant.

- A student has been previously told by a physician to cut down or stop drinking.

- A student currently has a medical condition that is exacerbated by alcohol (e.g., ulcers, diabetes).

In the latter two instances, we always defer to medical specialists to determine whether or not any degree of alcohol use is advisable, in light of a student's medical history. Students in such cases are encouraged to abstain until they can arrange a medical consultation with their primary care physician.

Using Computer-Generated Graphic Feedback

We recommend that the salient components of the feedback be summarized for each student graphically. An example of a graphic feedback sheet we have used is given in Appendix B of this manual (see Figure B.3 there). This graphic provides a student with personalized feedback about his or her pattern of alcohol use compared to the actual norms for other college students, and it overviews the student's risks for alcohol problems. The graphic is designed in such a way that it can stand on its own, although we recommend that a therapist review all categories in the graphic with a student.

There are several benefits of utilizing graphic feedback. A graphic feedback sheet can serve as an outline for the session, particularly given the extent of information to be covered. Second, use of the graphic can aid in building rapport as the therapist and student "examine" the content of the graphic together. The intention here is for the therapist and student to sit side by side (both literally and figuratively), sorting through the data and making sense of them together. This may be similar to a traveler and guide examining a map together to chart out their course. Third, in our experience, students like to receive visual graphics. A student typically "perks up" and takes more interest when a therapist pulls out a personalized graphic feedback sheet that summarizes information provided during the assessment. Finally, the student gets to take the graphic home for future use and reference.

The production of graphics for feedback can be costly and may require expensive computer expertise and equipment. Several options are available for generating this level of personalized feedback. Assessment information can be entered into a data base program such as Microsoft Access (either manually or with a scanner), and then can be read from a graphics program into a graphics template to generate the actual personalized feedback. This is the kind of system we used for generating the graphic feedback sheet depicted in Figure B.3 of Appendix B. The primary limitation of this approach is the inability to program complex decision rules about the data and to incorporate a complex algorithm for personalized messages.

A second method for generating personalized feedback involves the use of sophisticated computer programs capable of unlimited "if–then" decision rules about the data, as well as personalized messages. We have recently developed a multimedia computerized assessment program that automatically generates personalized graphic feedback capable of 2,443,000 different responses. This program, called Multi-Media Assessment of Student Health (MMASH; see Dimeff, 1996), was originally developed for use within a primary care setting, with student health center physicians and nurses providing a brief intervention aided by the MMASH personalized graphic feedback. Using headphones, students receive instructions in how to use the program through narration, then input their answers directly into a computer with a mouse and keyboard. Once complete, the personalized feedback is printed out immediately by a printer attached to the computer.

Developing a Personalized Blood Alcohol Level Chart and Card

Following the initial interview, we construct a personalized blood alcohol level (BAL) chart and a smaller, wallet-sized laminated BAL card for each student. The chart provides an approximation of a student's BAL over time after consuming alcoholic beverages, and is adjusted for the weight and sex of the individual. Figure 5.1 is an example of a BAL chart. BAL calculations for men and women of different weights are available in Matthews and Miller (1979).

NUMBER OF HOURS

NUMBER OF DRINKS	0 HOURS	1 HOUR	2 HOURS	3 HOURS	4 HOURS	5 HOURS	6 HOURS	7 HOURS	8 HOURS	9 HOURS	10 HRS
1	.025	.009	0	0	0	0	0	0	0	0	0
2	.051	.035	.019	.003	0	0	0	0	0	0	0
3	.077	.061	.045	.029	.013	0	0	0	0	0	0
4	.103	.087	.071	.055	.039	.023	.007	0	0	0	0
5	.129	.113	.097	.081	.065	.049	.033	.017	.001	0	0
6	.155	.139	.123	.107	.091	.075	.059	.043	.027	.011	0
7	.181	.165	.149	.133	.117	.101	.085	.069	.053	.037	.021
8	.206	.190	.174	.158	.142	.126	.110	.094	.078	.062	.046
9	.232	.216	.200	.184	.168	.152	.136	.120	.104	.088	.072
10	.258	.242	.226	.210	.194	.178	.162	.146	.130	.114	.098
11	.284	.268	.252	.236	.220	.204	.188	.172	.156	.140	.124
12	.310	.294	.278	.262	.246	.230	.214	.198	.182	.166	.150
13	.336	.320	.304	.288	.272	.256	.240	.224	.208	.192	.176
14	.362	.346	.330	.314	.298	.282	.266	.250	.234	.218	.202
15	.387	.371	.355	.339	.323	.307	.291	.275	.259	.243	.227
16	.413	.397	.381	.365	.349	.333	.317	.301	.285	.269	.253
17	.439	.423	.407	.391	.375	.359	.343	.327	.311	.295	.279
18	.465	.449	.433	.417	.401	.385	.369	.353	.337	.321	.305
19	.491	.475	.459	.443	.427	.411	.395	.379	.363	.347	.331
20	.517	.501	.485	.469	.453	.437	.421	.405	.389	.373	.357

FIGURE 5.1. Sample blood alcohol level (BAL) chart, showing BAL as a function of number of drinks and time for a male weighing about 145 pounds. A drink is any beverage that contains 1/2 ounce of ethyl alcohol.

Providing a "Tips" Sheet

In addition to the personalized graphic feedback sheet and the BAL chart and card, students are provided with a generic "tips" sheet that summarizes information about alcohol and its effects, highlighting the main points discussed during the second session. Lists and graphics are used to illustrate various concepts (e.g., effects on people without tolerance to alcohol at different BALs, the biphasic response to alcohol). The "tips" sheet also includes basic alcohol skills training information and moderation strategies, such as spacing alcoholic drinks further apart, drinking for quality instead of for quantity, alternating alcoholic beverages with nonalcoholic beverages, drinking beer rather than hard alcohol, and setting a drinking limit. Finally, the sheet can include additional information about alcohol to grab students' attention, such as the amount of money spent by the alcoholic beverage industry to promote its products on college campuses. Figures B.5 and B.7 in Appendix B are examples of "tips" sheets we have used.

THE ACTUAL MEETING

This section reviews the full content of the second session of BASICS. The description of content we give here is based on our research protocol. Our account of the clinical process, our notes of caution, and our other comments are products of having conducted hundreds of these brief interventions within the context of our clinical work, and of having spent many more hours training others to administer this intervention. We begin with some preliminary remarks about how best to orient the student to this second session, and some general comments about clinical process.

Orienting, Reestablishing Rapport, and Strengthening Commitment

The overarching goal of this second session is to provide the student with the motivation and skills to reduce negative consequences stemming from the use of alcohol, by providing the student with feedback based on the initial session and other information that will propel the student in the direction of change. More specific features of this broad goal include the following components:

1. Providing the student with specific feedback about his or her pattern of drinking and risks associated with drinking.

2. Furnishing psychoeducational information about alcohol that will assist the student to make more informed and less risky decisions about how to drink alcohol.

3. Providing advice and recommendations about modifications to the current pattern of use, at a level commensurate with the student's current stage of readiness to change.

4. Building student's motivation and commitment to change.

5. Assisting in the removal or reduction of barriers or obstacles to change.

Although the therapist has provided the student with a general panorama of the brief intervention at the beginning of the first session, it is nonetheless important that the therapist take a few minutes to orient the student to the terrain of the second session, as well as to permit the therapist and student to become reacquainted. Dialogue 5.1 gives one example of how the therapist might orient the student to this session. Notice that in addition to orienting the student, the therapist also works to reestablish the student's commitment to engage in the brief intervention by eliciting feedback about the agenda ("How does that sound?") and inviting the student to add further topics to the session's agenda.

Dialogue 5.1. Orienting the Student to the Second Session

THERAPIST: Welcome back! As you know, this is probably our last session, unless we decide for whatever reason to meet again. We can discuss that later. For now, I just want to take a minute to go over what I had planned for this session, and to see if there is anything else you had in mind that you want to put on the table for our meeting today.

STUDENT: Okay.

THERAPIST: Since the last time we met, I've put together the information that you provided during our first meeting into this graphic, which will allow us to take a closer look at how you drink in comparison to your peers and at some risks that may be associated with your drinking. We'll start by taking a look at your monitoring cards, then move into taking a closer look together at this graphic information. We'll then spend a bit of time talking about how you might make use of this information in the future. I should also mention that throughout our meeting, I'll be discussing some basic points about alcohol—some of which you may already know, and some of which will be quite new. How does that sound?

STUDENT: Yeah, that sounds okay. That graphic looks pretty interesting.

THERAPIST: Good. The graphic is kind of interesting, in that it allows us to look at a lot of information at once. Now is there anything else you also want to make sure we cover or discuss today that you'd like to add to the agenda?

STUDENT: No, not really. Oh, yeah, I would be interested in knowing if there's a problem in using alcohol at the same time as smoking pot.

THERAPIST: Good question. Okay, we'll add that to our list. Anything else you want to make sure we discuss?

TABLE 5.1. Components of Second Session and Approximate Time Lengths

Basic topics for feedback and advice session (in order of general use)	Approximate time length
Orientation and recommitment	3–5 minutes
Review and discussion of monitoring cards	5–7 minutes
Review of drinking pattern with comparison against norms	7–10 minutes
Review of personal risks and negative consequences	7–10 minutes
Advice and recommendations	7–10 minutes
Generalizing use of strategies beyond the brief intervention	3–8 minutes

STUDENT: No, that's it.

THERAPIST: All right. So why don't we get started? Now I want you to feel free to stop me to ask a question or to clarify something. I want to make this as interactive and helpful to you as possible.

STUDENT: Okay, I can do that.

We wish to make the following additional points about the structure of the second session, prior to getting started with our review. Table 5.1 lists the major topics of Session 2 in the order we most commonly use, as well as the approximate length of time we devote to each component, based on a 50-minute-session. We emphasize again that there is nothing "magic" about this particular ordering, although we have found it useful and convenient. In addition, psychoeducational material and topic-specific advice and recommendations can be inserted at any point where these are clinically relevant to the discussion at hand. As Table 5.1 indicates, it is necessary to move through the second session swiftly if one is to get through the basic components of this session in the time allotted.

Clinical Process and Approach to Providing Feedback and Advice

Unlike the fairly structured first session, the second session requires a great deal more flexibility. The therapist must move quickly and speedily—in a sense, "pulling" the student along just enough to enhance motivation, but not so much so that the student becomes annoyed or resistant. Although experience is nothing less than a wonderful teacher, we have found certain strategies helpful in increasing our overall effectiveness. We have found it useful to keep the following "rules of thumb" in our minds as we approach the brief intervention:

- Take a pragmatic realist's stance.

- Avoid "shoulds."

- Motivation and insight are not always required for behavior to change.

- "Quantum" change can occur.

- Get **specific** commitments for **behavioral action steps** from the student, when possible.

The first rule of thumb is to search for and find a synthesis[1] between **pragmatic realism and** *quantum change.*[2] As much as we may want to eradicate all risk, we should first have realistic expectations for what is possible to achieve as a result of the brief intervention, and then seek to maximize its impact and strive for quantum change. Taking a pragmatic realist's stance includes not assuming that a student will be interested in making changes in his or her drinking habits by the end of the brief intervention, and remembering that the decision is ultimately the student's to make. The harder a therapist pushes his or her position, the more likely the student is to close the door and not "hear" the message the therapist is trying to impart. In our experience, the ability to generate creative solutions and advice for students tailored to their goals or needs is directly related to the ability to hear students' descriptions of what's important to them. We have found that thinking like a pragmatic realist firmly rooted in harm reduction principles opens doors and makes options available, as opposed to funneling all students down the same chute, in the same direction, and on the same course.

Although it is effective in many respects to take a pragmatic realist's stance, it is also equally important to "aim high" by holding out hope that big-change steps can be facilitated within the context of a brief intervention. Striving for high goals, as opposed to lowering the ceiling for a given student on the basis of what he or she says or reports about his or her interest in change, is important if the maximum therapeutic effect is to be achieved. Here is where it is particularly useful to recognize that quantum change does (and therefore, can) occur. This dialectical position, which maintains two apparently opposite positions at once, will further contribute to the speed and overall effectiveness of the brief intervention.

The second rule of thumb is to avoid "should"-ing the student. Because young adults have often been critically judged by older adults for previous lifestyle decisions (or

---

[1]The first author wishes to acknowledge the contribution of Marsha M. Linehan and her theory of Dialectical Behavior Therapy (DBT) in offering a behavior therapy approach for transforming polar-opposite positions (thesis = pragmatic realism; anti-thesis = quantum realism) into a coherent synthesis that is comprised of the spirit of each position as well as the tension and conflict that exists between them).

[2]The concept of **quantum change** is a term recently coined by William Miller, PhD, to describe a not-so-uncommon experience reported by individuals who suddenly and profoundly change in some important way. In contrast to the principles of shaping, where an individual progresses incrementally in a step-wise fashion toward a particular behavior, quantum change refers to radical behavioral change similar to a sudden metamorphosis. While anecdotal examples are not uncommon (e.g., the smoker who after 30 years one day stopped all use of tobacco products after the birth of his child; the obese individual who seldom exercised throughout her life began a rigorous and regular exercise program on a daily basis which she sustained throughout the remainder of her life; the suicidal and self-harming individual who one day ceased all suicidal and self-harm behaviors because of a profound spiritual experience), the behavior change literature has only recently begun reflecting such experiences.

perceive that they have been critically judged), acting in a fashion that conveys such a judgment can result in students' "shutting down" or simply going along with the program and communicating interest when they have no intention of thinking about, let alone using, the content from the intervention. The more willing and able a student is to convey open, honest reactions to the feedback and advice, the more able the therapist will be to weave this information into a meaningful plan, thereby increasing the likelihood that the student will try out new harm reduction behaviors.

Third, it is important to know that motivation or insight is not always required as a condition for behavior to change. One example of this, discussed in Chapter 4, is the reactive effect of monitoring one's behavior. When a person monitors a particular behavior, the behavior often changes—not as a result of the person's being more motivated to change, but as a result of increased awareness of a particular habit. A college student who drinks less in a particular context does not necessarily do so because he or she is motivated per se to drink less. Instead, the situational cues (e.g., playing softball on a Saturday afternoon with a group of high school friends) may simply result in lighter drinking. In fact, most behaviors are learned, reinforced, and modified without a person's ever having any conscious awareness or intent of changing. This is particularly important in working with students who are difficult, and sometimes seemingly impossible, to motivate. Although much of BASICS is based on building interest and intent to change, this does not mean that we should not apply behavioral principles (e.g., shaping or modifying the context) that can result in behavioral changes without motivation.

The final rule of thumb pertains to getting specific commitments from a student. As previously described, having clients commit themselves to a particular activity increases the probability that the behavior will occur. Securing commitments can (and perhaps, in this context, should) be performed in a "light" fashion, and is very different from asking that a promise be made.

Providing Feedback and Advice

We now describe the actual provision of feedback and advice. A number of general "rules," suggested strategies for making particular comments and providing specific advice, and clinical highlights are incorporated throughout this discussion.

Reviewing Monitoring Card Homework

The second session typically begins with a review of the student's homework. We recommend that a therapist begin with the monitoring cards for several reasons. First, doing so acknowledges the student's efforts and willingness to honor his or her commitment with the therapist to participate actively in BASICS and to do the requested homework assignment. Second, a student is often just as excited about and interested in receiving feedback from a therapist as from a teacher. In a sense, the student enters into

• • •

the session expecting to receive something from the therapist (e.g., praise, feedback, etc.) for his or her work. Finally, reviewing the monitoring cards first imposes a structured and reasonably safe task, and thus serves as another means of reestablishing rapport.

Before attempting to extract the rich data that lie within the monitoring cards, a therapist should first provide the student with an opportunity to debrief the homework. We usually start by asking an open-ended question such as this:

"How did the monitoring go for you over the past 2 weeks?"

This also serves the purpose of providing the therapist with some sense of how (in)accurate the data are and of how much effort the student has exerted in completing the cards. Next, the therapist asks another open-ended question to elicit the perceived impact of the experience of monitoring for the student, and to determine how much the student thought about what he or she was were observing and recording. We generally ask a question such as this:

"Having now recorded your drinking behavior for the past 2 weeks, what did you notice or learn that you may not have realized before?"

We are specifically interested in what students have learned from monitoring their drinking. What did they notice? What did they learn? What became more clear as a result? Did they discover any surprises? What barriers did they encounter, if any, in monitoring their drinking? How well were they able to figure out solutions to the problems that presented themselves?

After the student has an opportunity to debrief the monitoring experience, the therapist begins focusing his or her efforts on the content yielded from the data. The student is first asked to describe what he or she has recorded. Typically, a student will orient the therapist to the cards, usually pointing out his or her heaviest-drinking days. We recommend that the therapist assume a collaborative and investigative stance with the student. That is, the therapist and the student look together at the cards, making sense of the data and extracting information from the cards about the pattern. The microscope's lens begins to focus on how often and how much the student drank, usually through a question like this one:

"Let's see. How many days did you actually drink alcohol? What amount did you average when you did drink?"

Once the typical and peak quantity and frequency of use are obtained, the therapist then gives the student a personalized BAL chart and teaches him or her how to estimate the approximate typical and peak BALs for the monitoring period.

To ascertain the peak BAL, the therapist can ask the student to recall the occasion during the period when he or she was most intoxicated. The student's peak intoxication experience can then be compared to approximate BALs. This process provides a forum to discuss how to calculate BALs, how much alcohol equals one standard drink, and what alcohol's effects are at different BALs, as well as to identify risks.

Depending on what unfolds in this discussion, the therapist may begin providing the student with additional psychoeducational information about alcohol. For example, a review of information about alcohol effects at different BALs for nontolerant persons often fits within the general discussion of monitoring cards. The therapist can ask the student to describe how he or she experienced the effects of alcohol on one of the recorded occasions. The therapist and student can then compare the student's alcohol effects on a particular occasion to the usual effects people without tolerance to alcohol experience. Should the student report that he or she did not "feel" the alcohol effects or had a much less robust response, this may open the way for a discussion of tolerance. **As tempting as it may be to provide all kinds of information to the student at this point, the therapist should avoid "lecturing" or otherwise bombarding the student with information about alcohol. The provision of skills training and information must always be tempered with the goal of increasing the student's motivation to change.**

Some of the richest data contained in the cards concern the specific situational factors associated with the student's use. Although we typically hold off on discussing the role of these contextual factors in heavy drinking until a bit later in the session, a therapist can nonetheless begin to highlight and name the factors associated with heavy use while talking through the card with the student. For example, the therapist might comment:

> "Hmm. It seems that you drank the heaviest on Saturdays, when you were at the tavern with your friends drinking shots. Is that consistent with your impression? (*Student*: 'Yeah, pretty much.') And it looks like on both occasions, you were in a pretty good mood, feeling relaxed and happy."

Generally speaking, information about the situational factors associated with drinking is usually accurate, even when the data about the quantity consumed are questionable. Students usually remember who they were with and where they were drinking, even if the cards were not completed for several days after the drinking occasion.

Providing Feedback on the Student's Drinking Pattern and Drinking Norms

After reviewing the monitoring cards and introducing the BAL chart, the therapist begins to provide feedback and advice. First, the therapist orients the student to the personalized graphic feedback sheet that summarizes the assessment materials. We encourage the therapist to take a few brief moments before moving into the actual feedback to do this. The therapist might make a transitional statement to orient the student to the move from reviewing the monitoring cards to the provision of feedback, such as the one given below:

"Let's see how the information you collected on the monitoring cards compares to the other information you provided the last time we met. This feedback sheet summarizes some of the information you and I discussed the last time we met. It also includes some information from the questionnaires you completed after our meeting. (*The therapist presents the graphic feedback sheet to the student.*) Notice that your drinking habits are summarized here on the left side, and personal risks associated with drinking alcohol are overviewed here on the right. Okay, so what I'd like to do now is go through this information with you. How does that sound? (*Student*: *'Fine.'*) Now as we go, please stop me along the way with any questions or comments that you might have about the material. Fair enough?"

The therapist then begins at the top of the graphic and moves down it, pausing along the way to elicit the student's reactions to the material, to highlight expressions and/or statements of concerns made by the student, and to answer questions that arise while providing the feedback. Information is first provided about the student's typical pattern of drinking, followed by a comparison of this pattern to general student norms. Feedback is then presented regarding the student's perception of typical drinking norms for college students.

Present Pattern of Use

The primary purpose of providing feedback about present consumption patterns is to increase students' awareness about how much and how frequently they consume alcohol. Information typically reviewed for this purpose is derived from the monitoring cards and from the typical and episodic portions of the Brief Drinker Profile (BDP). Specific topics include the student's frequency of use, average and peak quantity consumed on a weekly basis, BAL attained on an average occasion of drinking, and the highest (or peak) BAL reached during the assessment window.

As previously mentioned, we recommend that the therapist compare responses to drinking questions provided during the interview with answers to the drinking items in the questionnaire packet, to ensure accuracy of information. A final comparison is made with the data gathered from the monitoring cards. Information appearing on the graphic feedback is derived from the typical and episodic portions of the BDP. When discrepancies in significant details (e.g., drinking pattern, alcohol dependence, degree of problems resulting from alcohol use) emerge, we ask the student to clarify his or her responses during the second interview. We typically do this in a low-key way, like the television detective Columbo (scratching our heads and thinking out loud in an effort to make sense of both sets of details as true), in an effort to avoid putting a student too much on the spot while emerging with a clear picture of the student's behavior and risks.

Dialogue 5.2 illustrates a typical therapist–student interaction involving this feedback. Note that information is presented in a clear, straightforward fashion; in some cases, it is read directly from the personalized graphic feedback. Information that may be confusing—namely, the presentation of the percentile ranking—is described by the therapist in a couple of different ways to clarify and emphasize the point. Whenever possible, the student's behavior is compared to other common markers, such as the state's legal limit for driving under the influence of alcohol (in the case of the BAL feedback) and actual college norms (in the case of the student's pattern of drinking and perception of college norms). Consistent with the strategies of motivational interviewing, the therapist highlights the student's reactions or concern about the feedback, in an effort to increase the student's own awareness of or interest in change.

Dialogue 5.2. Review of Student's Drinking Habits and Comparison to College Norms

THERAPIST: Okay, starting here in the upper left portion of the sheet, you reported that you typically drink on three to four occasions weekly, each time drinking between five and six drinks.

STUDENT: Yeah, that's about average, I'd say.

THERAPIST: When we compare how often and how much you typically drink to other undergraduate university students, you place in the 97th percentile rank. That means that about 3% of all college undergrads drink more than you, and 97% drink less than you.

STUDENT: No way! Wow! 97%? Wow! (*Pause*)

THERAPIST: You seem quite surprised, like this wasn't what you expected.

STUDENT: That just seems really high!

THERAPIST: Next, we calculated the BAL that you typically reach when you drink, in addition to your highest BAL from the period of drinking we discussed before. These are BAL estimates based on your sex and weight. Your typical BAL was estimated at 0.17%, and your peak BAL was estimated at 0.295%. To put this into some kind of perspective, the Washington State limit is 0.08%.

STUDENT: Wow! I'm really up there. (*Pause*) No way. Could that be right? That just seems really high.

THERAPIST: It is based on an estimate of what your BAL would be, given your pattern of drinking before the homecoming football game. You're right. It is high. (*Pause*) Usually we don't see BALs as high as your peak.

STUDENT: I can't get over that! When can you die from alcohol poisoning?

THERAPIST: That's a good question. Typically, things get increasingly dangerous at around 0.30% BAL. You were pretty close to that level.

STUDENT: I can't get over this. Even my typical pattern is almost twice the legal limit, huh?

THERAPIST: Right. It's close. Let's go on to the next area here. You indicated that you believe the typical college student drinks close to what you do—about three to four times a week, and about five to six drinks per occasion. As it turns out, the typical university student at the University of Washington drinks considerably less: about once or twice weekly, and between six and eight drinks total for the week.

STUDENT: I was off a little.

THERAPIST: Yeah. This also explains your surprise at your percentile ranking, doesn't it?

STUDENT: Yeah. I just assumed that most people were like me and my friends, you know?

THERAPIST: That's pretty common. We sort of assume that other people are like us when it comes to certain habits. If you and your friends drink a lot, you sort of end up with a notion that what really isn't average seems average.

Situational Factors

After the student's drinking pattern is reviewed, situational factors are then identified to determine the contexts in which heavy drinking occurs. Sources for this information include the interview (discussions of any occasions where the individual had more to drink than the typical pattern) and the monitoring cards. The primary aim in discussing the contextual factors is simply to identify what they are, not necessarily to "do" anything with this information at this point. The therapist can provide a rationale for attending to these factors, if appropriate:

> "The decision to drink—or drinking heavily, for that matter—seldom occurs within a vacuum, but is usually influenced by external or situational factors. If you think about it for a minute, you'll probably notice that there are some similarities about the occasions when you drink heavily. For example, you are with a particular group of friends, or it's a particular day or evening of the week. Maybe you're engaging in a particular activity, like partying."

The therapist might next elicit this information from the student before turning to written sources of information:

> "Generally speaking, where do you do most of your heavy drinking, and who are you with?"

The therapist can highlight the specific contextual factors that emerged from the episodic portion of the BDP and the monitoring cards. The therapist might then ask the student whether he or she can think of any other contributing factors not already reviewed. We have found that place of drinking, beverage consumed, and the presence of certain "drinking friends" are often the most salient situational factors. Other factors likely to be overlooked include the following:

- Academic quarter (more drinking occurs in the fall and spring quarters).

- Midterm and final examinations.

- Special school or sporting events (e.g., football game with university rivals, etc.).

Although the reason for discussing this information is usually not made explicit at this point in the session, the obvious reason is to provide a basis for making specific recommendations for moderation. To the extent that drinking behavior is situationally determined, individuals can decide to "tweak" some aspects of their behavior in a particular situation to prevent heavy drinking. We will return to this point later when discussing specific moderation strategies.

Perceptions of Norms and Percentile Ranks

The primary aim of feedback about norms and percentile ranks is to place the student's drinking within a broader context of college student drinking habits—both to provide a basis for comparison, and to raise the student's awareness of what actually **is** a typical pattern of drinking for students. In our original research, three kinds of feedback were provided:

1. We first compared each student's typical frequency and quantity of drinking to student norms.

2. Each student's drinking pattern was then converted into a percentile rank, which provided another means of comparison.

3. Finally, we compared each student's perceptions of college student norms to the actual norms. (We have recently incorporated an additional comparison in our clinical work with students: norms for adult women and men residing in the United States. This demonstrates that what is "normal" or "average" for college students far exceeds what is typical for adults in general. Patterns for students who appear in the "typical" or "below-average" range for college students end up being above average when compared across the board to these adult samples.)

The normative data used in our original research were derived from previous studies conducted by our center on undergraduate drinking patterns at the University of Washington. On the average, undergraduates at the University of Washington typically drink alcohol on one to two occasions weekly, and consume between three and four drinks per occasion. Students who consume between six and eight drinks a week are in the 50th percentile, suggesting that there are just as many college students who drink more as who drink less than this.

Dialogue 5.3 illustrates the therapist providing this feedback to a male student who significantly exceeds the college drinking norm (by 16 drinks per week), but who believes that his drinking level is somewhat lower than the college average. The therapist first observes the student's typical pattern and the student's perceived norms for college drinking, then provides the percentile feedback. Notice how the therapist emphasizes the salient numbers in several different ways while making the same point. Notice also that the therapist neither exaggerates nor softens the data's impact, but instead highlights the data and amplifies only those reactions expressed by the student.

Dialogue 5.3. Providing Feedback on Drinking Pattern, Perceived Norms, and Percentile Ranking

THERAPIST: As we have already discussed somewhat, you usually consume about 24 beers on three different occasions in an average week. Earlier we asked you to estimate how much the typical college student drinks in a week. You guessed about 28 drinks a week. That would make your drinking pattern slightly lower than the typical college pattern. As it turns out, the actual average for college students is considerably lower than you imagined, and is also much lower than your average. The average is about once or twice weekly, and about three to four drinks per occasion for an average total of six to eight drinks per week. (*Pause*) As you can see, that's significantly less than you had originally suspected. You are drinking about 16 drinks more per week than the typical student. That's about 64 drinks a month.

STUDENT: Wow. That seems really high.

THERAPIST: Well, yes, it is rather high. You seem quite surprised by those numbers. It wasn't what you expected, was it?

STUDENT: No, not at all. Most of my friends tease me about being a lightweight. Wow . . .

THERAPIST: It sounds like your friends drink quite a bit more than you. Is that right?

STUDENT: I don't know if I'd say "quite a bit more," but they do drink more than me. Yeah.

THERAPIST: It's not uncommon for groups of friends to have similar drinking habits. If a person's friends drink a lot, they too are more likely to drink heavily. For that reason, it's not uncommon for people who are actually among the heaviest drinkers in college to have an idea that their drinking is no different from that of most college students, when in fact it's quite different.

STUDENT: Yeah, that makes sense.

THERAPIST: The next number here is your percentile rank for your typical drinking pattern, again compared to other college students. It's sort of a quick way of making sense of this information we collected about how much and how frequently you drink. When we look at the total number of drinks you consume per week, compared to other students, your pattern falls in the 96th percentile bracket. That means that only 4% of college students drink more than you, and about 96% report drinking less than you do. (*Pause for student response*)

STUDENT: No way. (*Student studies graphic's figures*)

THERAPIST: Again, it seems like the figure is much higher than you suspected. Is that so?

STUDENT: Yeah. That's really high . . . that's *really* high. We look like a bunch of losers or something.

THERAPIST: It's really surprising to you to see just how different your pattern of drinking is compared to other students, isn't it?

STUDENT: Yeah. Wow. I keep going back to that number—96!

Heavy-drinking students typically react with more surprise and concern to these data than to any other feedback presented. Although some challenge the accuracy of the norms we use for this comparison, others offer specific explanations for how they (and their friends) may drink more than most but are not afflicted by alcohol problems. Still others respond with concerned amazement and disbelief, unaware that their drinking is so far out of the "normal" range.

Occasionally, students have attempted to challenge the validity of the normative data by reasoning that most college students would underestimate their amount of alcohol use when completing a questionnaire for university researchers. These students typically respond:

> "I don't see how those figures can be accurate. They seem way too low. Almost everyone that I know drinks way more than the college average. The students who filled out your questionnaires probably don't tell the truth."

In these circumstances, we typically respond by indicating that although some students may attempt to falsify their report, the data from our studies (see Table 5.2) are generally consistent with national figures. This discussion also provides an opportunity to discuss how college students typically associate with persons with similar lifestyle habits, and how this sometimes makes it difficult for a student to get a good sense of what constitutes "typical" or "average" behavior across the spectrum of all college students.

TABLE 5.2. Percentile Rankings by Quantity of Alcohol Consumed Weekly: Data for University of Washington Undergraduates

Number of drinks consumed weekly	% of students who drink at least this amount
< 1 drink per week	90%
1 drink per week	82%
2 drinks per week	75%
3 drinks per week	65%
6 drinks per week	55%
8 drinks per week	46%
10 drinks per week	33%
13 drinks per week	20%
17 drinks per week	12%
20 drinks per week	9%
30 drinks per week	2%

Providing Feedback about Risks and Consequences Associated with Alcohol Use

Once the basic feedback about the student's drinking habits is reviewed, the direction of the session shifts to reviewing negative consequences from drinking. Most heavy-drinking students expect to "mature out" of their heavy-drinking habits after leaving college, and express little concern about long-term health effects. Included in this feedback is a review of the specific negative consequences of alcohol use a student has previously experienced, as well as an assessment of vulnerability to alcohol problems on the basis of the student's family history alcoholism, history of alcohol dependence, positive alcohol expectancies, and perception of risks. Our aim in providing this information is to make it meaningful and relevant. Although the feedback here focuses primarily on immediate and short-term risks, we nonetheless include some discussion of potential long-term risks and effects.

Alcohol-Related Behavioral Problems

The primary aim of providing feedback about consequences is to help the student link past unwanted, embarrassing, or terribly problematic behaviors and experiences that occurred during or following heavy drinking with the heavy drinking itself. To the extent to which the best predictor of future behavior is past behavior, the therapist reviews these past experiences with the student and attempts to tie them directly to the degree of intoxication. In some cases, negative outcomes occur when students are mildly "buzzed." More likely than not, problems occur under conditions of extreme intoxication. This approach conveys the message that what is problematic is alcohol intoxication, and not necessarily drinking alcohol in general. We have found that students are generally more receptive to this approach, which for some will stand in contrast to messages they have received in the past from health professionals who favor the "Just Say No" approach over a message of moderation.

The first step in addressing the link between negative consequences and heavy drinking is to enter into a discussion with the student about the student's own perceptions of the ways in which alcohol has negatively affected his or her life or has resulted in specific problems. The therapist might pose the following question to the student:

> "From your perspective, in what ways, if any, has alcohol gotten in the way for you or resulted in unpleasant experiences?"

The therapist follows up this question by obtaining a general description of the student's degree of intoxication (e.g., "pretty buzzed," "really ripped," etc.) when the negative outcomes occurred. The therapist might ask:

> "In general, how intoxicated were you when you experienced these unwanted outcomes? Would you say you were, for example, not very drunk at all, or really drunk?"

> "Sometimes students report having different kinds of negative experiences at different stages or degrees of intoxication. Thinking back on your own experiences, I wonder if you've noticed a pattern yourself about the difference in the kinds of negative experiences you have when you are, say, lightly buzzed versus when you are much more intoxicated."

Within the context of our research, students were then provided feedback about the negative consequences they reported on the Rutgers Alcohol Problems Inventory (RAPI; White & Labouvie, 1989). Items summarized on the graphic feedback included all positively endorsed RAPI items pertaining to alcohol dependence (regardless of the frequency of occasions the student endorsed these) and RAPI items with the highest frequency of endorsement, up to a total of five problems listed. To begin this review, the therapist might state the following:

> "One of the surveys you completed asked you a number of questions about negative consequences you had from alcohol in the past 6 months. I've summarized some of these that you originally mentioned here on the graphic. You noted, for example, often getting into fights and embarrassing other people as a result of drinking alcohol."

The therapist then reads all items listed on the graphic out loud, pausing briefly after each item to provide an opportunity for the student to comment if he or she so desires. More often than not, students generally either sit quietly through this portion or offer an explanation for why they endorsed a particular item. It is important for the therapist to resist arguing with a student over the significance or severity of a particular item, particularly if the student is attempting to minimize its import. The point of assuming this position is to minimize the likelihood of increasing the student's defensiveness or psychological reactance, particularly when the student is in the precontemplative or contemplative stage of change. In fact, the therapist may sometimes want to align with the student when the student offers a reasonable explanation for endorsement of a particular item:

"I can see your point on that one. This item really doesn't fit that well for you in that context."

Positive Alcohol Expectancies

The aim of providing feedback about expectancies is threefold:

1. To increase the student's awareness of his or her implicit beliefs about alcohol, which may contribute to risky drinking.

2. To challenge the myth that alcohol effects are caused solely by the physiological properties of the alcohol, and thus to encourage consideration of psychological factors.

3. To encourage the student to experiment with psychological factors when drinking, so as to get the desired effects with less alcohol. In this sense, the therapist challenges the student to rely on the psychological cues rather than the alcohol to achieve the positive effects.

In advance of the interview, up to five positive outcome alcohol expectancies from the Comprehensive Effects of Alcohol (CEA) survey are summarized on the graphic feedback form. As previously mentioned, the therapist can identify these specific items by locating the CEA items that the student has endorsed as both pleasurable and likely to result from drinking. The therapist again begins by eliciting information from the student about the positive effects he or she expects to derive from drinking alcohol:

"What are the positive experiences you expect to get when you drink alcohol?"

Previously endorsed items from the CEA are then reviewed. After this review, the discussion then shifts to understanding the nature of the student's expectancies. Specifically, are they due to the pharmacological properties of alcohol, to psychological factors, or to both? The interviewer might ask:

"How do you account for these effects? Do you think that they come about as a result of the chemical properties from the alcohol, or for some other reason?"

The student is then introduced to the balanced-placebo design and the related body of research. (A review of this literature has been presented in Chapter 3 of this manual.) Often we will sketch the design for students and provide an explanation for each cell as we go. In reviewing this model, we emphasize both the importance of one's mental set and the environmental setting in contributing to the pleasurable alcohol effects, in addition to the pharmacological effects of alcohol. We also encourage students to conduct their own "Think–Drink" experiment (Rohsenow & Marlatt, 1981), to determine how they can maximize the positive psychological effects either without drinking alcohol at all or when drinking alcohol in moderate amounts.

We want to caution and alert the therapist new to BASICS to the temptation that frequently arises at this point—to slip into a lecturing mode, rather than maintaining the interactive, collaborative approach we have recommended earlier. This tendency is almost unavoidable in light of time constraints and the complexity of the model, not to mention its importance. The problem with this approach is that unless a therapist is unusually engaging and witty, the student may get bored or resent the unsolicited lecture.

We have found it helpful to elicit parallel real-world examples either from a student's own experiences (e.g., a prank played on a group of friends by the student) or from experiences common to other young people. For example, one student mentioned that when he was in high school, he and a friend told a group of students that they'd spiked the punch at their school dance when they actually hadn't. Within a short period of time, word spread, and students were flocking to the punch bowl. Meanwhile, the pranksters watched with amusement as their friends acted intoxicated, as if they really had consumed alcohol (e.g., acting disinhibited, some stumbling, etc.). Another student recalled an occasion when he and his friends had been drinking at a park one evening and became "pretty drunk." On the way home, they were stopped by a police officer for driving without their headlights on. Despite their drunken behavior at the park just minutes earlier, "we all sobered up" as the officer approached the car. In light of the information on alcohol expectancies, he realized that some of the drunken behavior was psychologically induced.

On occasion, a student will balk at the idea that psychological effects make such an important contribution to his or her pleasure while drinking. Understanding the nature of the student's skepticism is obviously an important step in cognitively challenging the student's beliefs. One common concern is that the student will have less fun or will feel left out if he or she drinks less. It is important to address this concern directly by emphasizing that the goal here is to help the student have fun without having to pay a high price for it. For students who express concern about peer pressure to drink or fears of feeling left out, we focus on problem-solving solutions to these awkward and difficult occasions. Seldom do students explicitly request information or assistance; for this reason, the therapist must listen carefully to pick up the specific concerns and to detect openness for help.

A second issue a student may raise involves questioning the relevance of psychological effects when alcohol is consumed heavily. This is a somewhat trickier issue to address. The student is right that as a person drinks more and the BAL rises, he or she will experience very specific behavioral experiences that are directly due to the drug effects of alcohol. Motor coordination, like cognitive capabilities, become impaired. However, the chemical properties of alcohol do not alone account for the experience and nullify the contribution of psychological effects; one set of effects doesn't "undo" or "outdo" the other in significance. In addition to the drug effects in the case of someone who is considerably intoxicated, the individual's prior experiences will also influence his or her experience through the principles of learning and conditioned response. It is for this reason that alcohol expectancies will vary for the same person from context to context, and that they may play a stronger role in one setting than in another.

Concern about Drinking and Perceived Risk for Alcohol Problems

We often find that heavy-drinking college students perceive their future risk of experiencing alcohol-related problems or unwanted negative consequences as considerably lower than one would expect on the basis of their past behavior. Furthermore, it is not uncommon for heavy-drinking college students to express relatively little interest in changing, or motivation to change, their drinking. Both dimensions are examined during the initial assessment, for these purposes: (1) to give the therapist some sense of how the student may respond to the feedback, and (2) to raise the student's awareness of how well his or her risk perceptions and motivation to change the current pattern of heavy drinking correspond to the actual risks for negative consequences from drinking.

This feedback is particularly useful in a case where there is a large disparity between the student's perceived and actual risk. In these instances, this feedback provides the student with an opportunity to step back and view the situation more critically or objectively. With respect to the goal of advancing the student through the stages of change, it provides an additional means for the therapist to assist the student in moving from precontemplation to contemplation. For a student whose perceptions of risk and concern are commensurate to the actual risks, this feedback can lead into a discussion of specific steps to take, thereby moving the student into the action stage.

The therapist can begin this portion of the feedback by reminding the student of the series of questions he or she completed about the likelihood of experiencing a series of unpleasant consequences or negative outcomes as a result of drinking. After providing the specific feedback on perceived risks, the therapist should then provide the feedback from the questions on the student's motivation to change. Ideally, the therapist attempts to tie these two discrete sets of data together into a cohesive clinical picture. As always, the therapist attends to the student's response to the feedback, eliciting his or her reactions and concerns. An example of how to begin providing this feedback is given below:

> "We asked you a series of questions about the extent to which you consider your drinking risky and whether you had considered changing how you drink before meeting with me today. It appears that when you completed the questionnaires, your perception of your risk was relatively low. In other words, you didn't seem to see yourself getting into any difficulties or having any problems because of your drinking. Not surprisingly, it appears you didn't feel a need to change how you

drink. I'm wondering how you feel now in light of some of the information we have reviewed."

In a case where the perception of risk is high and the interest in minimizing that risk is also high, the therapist might state the following:

"Judging from the questionnaires you completed the last time we met, it appears that you have a reasonably good sense about risks associated with your drinking and an interest in receiving some information that might help address these issues. Is that a fair reading of how you see things?"

Family History of Problem Drinking and/or Alcoholism

The aim of providing family history feedback is to alert students to their risk of developing alcohol problems as a function of genetic predisposition. Based on the number of blood relatives with alcohol problems, students are told that their risk is "negative," "positive," or "strongly positive." We have found that students typically show one of two extreme reactions to this information: Either they assign more power and significance to genetic factors than would be warranted on the basis of the research, or they dismiss this information altogether. It is important that the therapist not make the same mistake of either amplifying the significance of this information or dismissing the role of genetics completely.

The therapist can begin this portion of the feedback by reminding the student that a positive family history is simply one additional risk factor, and should not be interpreted as a forecast of the future. Just as an individual with a negative family history is not **necessarily immune** to developing alcohol problems, the student with a positive family history is not **necessarily destined** to meet the same fate as his or her relatives. Indeed, some studies have found that college students without family histories of alcoholism often have more problems with alcohol than family-history-positive students (Alterman, 1988; Alterman, Bridges, & Tarter, 1986; Baer et al., 1992).

The therapist can introduce this topic as follows:

"In this next area of feedback, we indicated your degree of risk for alcohol problems resulting from your family's history of difficulties with alcohol. During the first meeting, you indicated that your father had a period of excessive drinking when you were in your early teens. You also indicated that your mother has conveyed concern about your maternal grandfather's drinking. From what you gathered from her, it would appear that he too had difficulty with alcohol at one point during his life, right? I've assessed your risk stemming from this family history as positive. This does not mean that you necessarily have or will develop alcohol problems. This is simply one additional risk factor, which does nevertheless contribute to your overall risk configuration. Any questions about this?"

Another approach is to focus on the meaning of genetic heritability for the student, as illustrated in this example:

> "We really don't know at this time what the precise mechanism for heritability is. It could be that genetic factors influence a person's sensitivity to alcohol. It may have all to do with influencing personality style. We really don't know at this time. What does it mean for you?"

Although the focus of family history assessment within the context of our research was on genetic risk, and our coding of family history was applied uniformly to all participants, there is no reason why strict adherence to this particular focus needs to be maintained when BASICS is applied clinically. More specifically, a discussion about how and in what ways the student has experienced a family member's excessive drinking may produce a more fruitful conversation than a discussion of genetic risks. For example, if a student presents with a history of early family turmoil resulting from his or her stepfather's excessive and highly problematic drinking, not considering this as vital information in understanding the family's contribution to the student's risk (as a result of modeling or social learning) simply because the stepfather is not a blood relative would be an omission of valuable feedback about risk and acknowledgment of the importance of these experiences.

Indices of Alcohol Dependence

The three aims governing our review of indices of alcohol dependence are as follows:

1. To provide students with feedback about the extent to which they manifest symptoms of alcohol dependence.

2. To lay the groundwork for a medical referral or more intensive treatment for individuals manifesting moderate to severe alcohol dependence.

3. To help students learn how to recognize signs of alcohol dependence in the future.

Specific items a student has endorsed during the first interview or on self-administered measures of alcohol dependence are listed on the graphic (e.g., increased tolerance, engaging in dangerous activities shortly after drinking alcohol, or drinking more than the student had intended or planned). We purposely avoid the use of classifying labels, such as **mildly dependent,** to prevent students from becoming defensive. We also use the word **indices** in the phrase "indices of alcohol dependence" on the graphic, as opposed to **symptoms,** to further avoid alienating students. Depending on a student's openness and receptivity to the feedback, the therapist can add, "This level is generally consistent with mild alcohol dependence."

Like the feedback about negative experiences, the feedback about indices of alcohol dependence often produces a variety of responses from students, ranging from surprise and concern to minimization. As is always the case, it is important not to "push" students toward some acceptance of how problematic and severe their drinking is, but instead to maintain a more detached, nonjudgmental tone of exploration. This is particularly important in cases where a student does genuinely appear to show signs of moderate to severe alcohol dependence, but appears unconcerned or unfazed.

Dialogue 5.4 illustrates providing this feedback to a heavy-drinking male student who might meet diagnostic criteria for mild dependence, but who does not view his symptoms of alcohol dependence as problematic or as causes for concern. Instead, he attempts to explain to the therapist that these experiences are not so unusual for a college student living in a fraternity. Note that the therapist is careful not to insist on a particular problem label, and does not push for the student to accept that he is more dependent on alcohol than he believes. Instead, she attempts to understand his experience and shifts the focus from a label of **alcohol dependence** back to thinking about personal risks. The therapist wraps up the alcohol dependence portion of the feedback, then focuses more specifically on the portion of this feedback that the student acknowledges—tolerance to alcohol (see Dialogue 5.5, below).

Dialogue 5.4. Providing Feedback on Alcohol Dependence

THERAPIST: The next risk factor indicated here (*pointing to the graphic feedback sheet*) is the indices of alcohol dependence. You endorsed that you had experienced the following items associated with alcohol dependence in the past 6 months: tolerance to alcohol, drinking more than you had originally planned, and spending a lot of time on alcohol-related activities—specifically, either preparing to drink, drinking, or recovering from drinking episodes.

STUDENT: Right. I remember saying that, but I don't think I'm addicted to alcohol. I mean, everyone has to drink more than they first did when they started drinking to get the same effect. It's not like I'm out there drinking alone. I drink with my friends at parties. I don't think that makes me an alcoholic!

THERAPIST: You're raising several really important points. Just because a person endorses these items, it doesn't make that person "alcohol-dependent" or an alcoholic. Like you, I'm not particularly interested in labels or in labeling you or anyone else "alcohol-dependent." I *am* interested in thinking more about this from a health or risk perspective, and my guess is that may be an important issue for you, too, yes? You raise a second important point, too: It's very difficult to understand a person's behavior outside the context it occurs in. You are clearly saying, "Look, I drink the same way a lot of other college students drink, and I don't have a problem!"

STUDENT: Yeah, that's it. I know we drink a lot; I know I drink a lot, but I don't see myself in any way being *dependent* on alcohol.

• • •

THERAPIST: Fair enough. You know, I'm wondering. What would that look like in your mind? What does a person act like or look like who is alcohol-dependent?

STUDENT: I don't know. Middle-aged, unemployed, no family or friends left. I don't know. Someone who's got it bad.

THERAPIST: I see. No wonder you wanted to make it clear to me that you aren't like that! I'm thinking more about dependence as being on a sort of continuum, with nonproblem use on one end, abuse of alcohol in the middle, and alcohol dependence at the other end. As it turns out, when people drink large amounts of alcohol, certain changes occur both psychologically and physically to accommodate to drinking heavily. This may not come as any surprise to you; we usually refer to this as "tolerance to alcohol." Have you heard about tolerance to alcohol in the past?

STUDENT: Yeah. Some guy came to our fraternity and went over a bunch of information on alcohol. I think he talked about tolerance.

THERAPIST: So you probably know that tolerance to alcohol is sort of a mixed bag. We'll come back to that in a minute. To finish up on alcohol dependence, it sounds like you have recently had some experiences with alcohol that can indicate alcohol dependence. However, as we have discussed, when we place these experiences within the broader context of your lifestyle, they may not mean the same thing as they might for someone else in a different context. You don't experience yourself as dependent on alcohol.

STUDENT: Right.

THERAPIST: Okay, so this is something to be aware of, but not overinterpret. Let's return to the topic of tolerance to alcohol.

Alcohol Tolerance

The discussion of tolerance to alcohol fits well within the general discussion of alcohol dependence. Because most people who drink on a regular basis have some degree of tolerance to alcohol, this discussion can provide a more benign route to discussing alcohol dependence. Many students view tolerance in positive terms (e.g., "I can drink more and not get sick," or "I can hold my alcohol better than most"). In some instances, being able to hold one's alcohol better than most is socially reinforced by peers, who seem to perceive tolerance as a sign of a person's strength or maturity. As previously mentioned, students learn that although tolerance lends itself to certain rewards (e.g., drinking more with fewer negative symptoms), it also diminishes the peak positive effects from alcohol, and it "costs" more (the biphasic response is reviewed in considerable detail below). From a health perspective, students are also taught that tolerance is usually a signal that people have blown past their bodies' natural warning signals that would normally inform them to slow the pace of their drinking, or to stop drinking altogether. Without these natural warning systems in place, individuals tend to drink more; in doing so they move further and further along the alcohol use continuum toward alcohol dependence.

One way of discussing this topic is to ask students to consider the number of drinks they require now to get a buzz from drinking alcohol, compared to when they first began drinking. We typically provide a brief explanation about tolerance and make the point that a high tolerance to alcohol is usually associated with alcohol dependence. For this reason, we encourage students to keep their tolerance to alcohol down by either drinking less or taking a vacation from heavy drinking for a several-week period. Dialogue 5.5 is a continuation of Dialogue 5.4 (the student is the one who resists the idea that he is alcohol-dependent).

Dialogue 5.5. Discussing Tolerance to Alcohol

THERAPIST: Let's go back to tolerance for a moment. Okay?

STUDENT: Yeah, sure.

THERAPIST: Okay. In comparison to other periods in your life, how tolerant to alcohol do you suppose you are right now?

STUDENT: I don't know. I am probably more tolerant. Definitely more tolerant compared to when I first started drinking. When I first began drinking, it hardly took more than a beer before I was feeling the effects. I was really a lightweight!

THERAPIST: Okay, so in comparison to when you first began drinking, you think you have a lot more tolerance. Now would you say that this is the most tolerant to alcohol you have ever been, or have there been other periods when you were more tolerant?

STUDENT: Well, I'd have to say that I had the most tolerance the summer before I started college. I was kicking around a lot with my friends, living on this ranch doing ranch, work all summer. We mostly drank. There wasn't much else to do.

THERAPIST: So, in comparison to then, your tolerance to alcohol has dropped.

STUDENT: Yeah.

THERAPIST: That's good from my perspective. See, tolerance is your body's way of adapting to the alcohol. It is sort of like your body's natural warning system alerting you that you've had enough to drink. The more people drink alcohol, the more they blow past this warning system that's telling them to slow down or stop drinking. The more this happens, the closer people come to being dependent or to having other health problems resulting from really heavy drinking. Does that make sense to you?

STUDENT: Yeah, I suppose.

THERAPIST: Unlike a lot of things in life, including liver damage from too many years of heavy drinking, tolerance is usually quite simple to reverse. For many people, it's not a permanent condition, as you know from your own experiences. Often when people don't drink at all for about a month, or they cut way back, they tend to notice getting more "kick" from a drink.

STUDENT: Yeah, right. I don't drink during swim season because I'm on the team. When I start drinking again after the session is completed, I have to be more careful about how much I drink. Otherwise, I end up looking like an idiot.

THERAPIST: Sounds like you've learned about this the hard way.

STUDENT: That's pretty much it. There's been a few times! Now I know that the only thing between me making a total, utter jerk out of myself at a party and me just having fun is my tolerance.

THERAPIST: You're raising an important point. You're saying, "Look, tolerance ain't so bad. In fact, it's saved me on occasion." That's the real bind. On the one hand, you are able to drink more without getting as intoxicated and acting like a "jerk." On the other hand, it can be really expensive having to drink more to get the same effect, plus you're placing more stress on your liver and other body organs as you blow past the warning signals that we spoke about earlier. Given the toll on a person's body, I usually recommend that people work to lower their tolerance, either entirely or to whatever extent they can.

STUDENT: It definitely is more expensive! I know that for certain.

THERAPIST: Let's do the math quickly. As we discussed earlier, most people who don't have tolerance to alcohol experience a mild buzz at around 0.05% BAL. You said earlier that you typically drink for 4 hours when you're at a party. According to this BAL card I made you for a 170-pound male, you would need approximately five drinks to reach this level over the course of 4 hours to get a mild buzz. Based on what you know yourself about your tolerance today, how many drinks would you need to drink over the course of 4 hours to get and sustain a mild buzz?

STUDENT: Probably twice that many, at least.

THERAPIST: Okay, and what does it cost for you to drink twice as many?

STUDENT: I usually only drink Red Hook ESB. A half rack usually costs me about $14.

THERAPIST: Okay, so half that would be about $7, right?

STUDENT: Right.

THERAPIST: So, on one average drinking occasion, tolerance ends up costing you about $7 per occasion. Okay, so if we consider the rest of the week and when you drink 4 times weekly use the same rate just as an example, you end up spending $28 more weekly, due to the current tolerance you've got built up. Over the course of the year, at 52 weeks per year, that's $1,456.

STUDENT: No way! I've never thought about it like that.

THERAPIST: Few people do. But when you do, it's sort of shocking, isn't it?

STUDENT: Indeed! I can't believe this.

In this discussion of alcohol tolerance, emphasis is placed on what is salient for the student—namely, the monetary expense incurred as a result of his tolerance. On the basis of his response to the alcohol dependence feedback, his lack of concern about the implications of tolerance for his health could be predicted. However, this student is not unlike many of his peers with respect to the salience of money. Once a modicum of interest in calculating the financial expense of his tolerance is expressed, the therapist in a sense "milks" this concern for all it's worth, through a series of specific calculations that clearly demonstrate the actual costs of tolerance over the course of a week and year.

Providing Feedback about General Lifestyle

In addition to providing feedback about the individual's use of alcohol, the therapist may choose to include a broader discussion of lifestyle factors and behaviors (e.g., stress and adjustment to university life, exercise, and diet) within the feedback session, using the other measures previously described. Specific feedback can center on the most salient aspect of the student's lifestyle. For example, living in a sorority may be the salient or primary lifestyle feature that exerts an influence over a number of specific lifestyle factors and health behaviors for a female student—from the setting in which the student drinks alcohol and eats meals, to how much alcohol and food she consumes, how much she studies and sleeps, and whether she practices protected sex. All feedback about specific lifestyle aspects can be presented within the broader context of living in a sorority, and the relationship between specific factors/behavior and the broader context can be examined. Other examples of broader contexts may include being affiliated with a particular sports team, living in a fraternity, identifying oneself as a young scholar with a perfect grade point average, being a member of a particular student organization (e.g., the lesbian, gay, and bisexual student union), and so forth.

Giving Advice and Making Recommendations

Contrary to the isolated placement of this topic at the end of this segment, we strongly suggest that the therapist make recommendations and give advice throughout the second session, wherever they naturally and appropriately "fit." Advice and recommendations provided early in the session are usually small in scope and related to a particular topic. For example, while discussing alcohol expectancies or the biphasic response, we often encourage students to put what we say to the test—either by focusing more deliberately on the setting and mental set while not drinking or drinking mildly, in the case of alcohol expectancies; or by finding their own point of diminishing return, in the case of the biphasic response to alcohol. Similarly, in cases where students indicate drinking a potentially lethal amount of alcohol or have medical conditions in which use of alcohol is contraindicated, advice to drink more moderately (in the first case) or to abstain altogether and consult a physician (in the second instance) is provided promptly. More general discussions about strategies to moderate drinking, or more broad-based discussion of specific, more intensive treatment recommendations, do usually occur at the end of the second session, after the therapist and student have had a chance to review the data together.

Although we recommend making certain suggestions to each student, much of the advice provided to students needs to be tailored to their specific needs and risks. As we have noted throughout this manual, it is important that advice be commensurate with both the student's readiness to use it and his or her actual level of risk. For example, recommending attendance at Alcoholics Anonymous for a student who has yet to recognize the severity of her or his pattern of use and negative consequences is likely to result not only in increased psychological reactance, but also in a loss of therapist credibility in the student's eyes. The ultimate result may be that the door to effective intervention and change is closed altogether.

Challenging the Student to a Field Experiment

Ideally, we like for students to leave the second session with specific plans or goals in mind for how they will apply BASICS in their lives. We encourage the therapist to be thinking throughout the second session about how this particular student might best begin integrating the materials and skills obtained. The question directed to the student can be as simple as "So what are you going to do with this information?" or "In light of this information, what makes sense? Honestly speaking, how do you see yourself making use of it?"

There is no "right" or "correct" answer to this question. The therapist's advice is only as good as the extent to it is tailored to the student's actual needs and to a realistic assessment of what the student will try following the intervention. For this reason, it is essential that the therapist avoid conveying any demands or "shoulds" for what the student "ought" to want to do. All efforts should instead be directed toward obtaining an honest response from the student. Accepting the student's expressed view of how he or she intends to make use of this intervention does **not** mean that the therapist should be resigned to accepting a student's lack of interest or limited interest in change. Acceptance simply means that the therapist should resist coaxing or cajoling the student to express an enthusiasm for change that he or she simply does not have (despite the therapist's efforts and desires) after receiving the feedback. In our experience, students will be forthcoming about their interest in change when therapists ask them about this without conveying "shoulds."

Encouraging students to conduct their own "field research" is one way to work advice giving into the conversation and to create a direct experience of bringing what the students have learned during the brief intervention to the specific contexts within their lives. They need to try on, experiment with, and learn new skills if they are to moderate their alcohol use successfully. It's important that in conducting such research, students pursue their experiments and interpret the findings in as unbiased a way as possible (rather than "discovering" what they set out to prove). Experiments could include the following:

- To what extent are the positive consequences students derive from drinking heavily due to the pharmacological effects of alcohol? To what extent are they psychological?

- How can students make use of the environmental setting and their mental set so as to get the most of the psychological effect from drinking? In other words, what contextual factors can they "tweak" to get the most out of drinking without drinking heavily?

- How do their friends use alcohol? Specifically, what might some of their friends' positive alcohol expectancies be, and what role does alcohol play in fulfilling the "magic elixir" prophecy?

Moderation Training

The most common advice we provide students is to moderate their drinking and to avoid binge drinking; accordingly, our most common recommendations are specific strategies in how to moderate drinking. Results from a recent methodological analysis of the alcohol treatment outcome literature (Miller, Brown, et al., 1995) indicate that more clinical studies of the effectiveness of moderation training (also known as **behavioral self-control training**) than of all other alcohol treatment approaches have been performed. These results further indicate that of all treatment approaches described in the literature, behavioral self-control training has the second largest number of positive findings. (For a further review of this literature, see Marlatt et al., 1993, and Hester, 1995.) Generally, studies have found that clients who are most successful with this approach tend to have a shorter history of alcohol problems and less severe dependence and problems (Hester, 1995).

A number of moderation training protocols are in existence. The ASTP (see Chapter 2), of which BASICS is one modality, uses a model similar to the one described in Miller and Munoz's (1982) self-help manual, *How to Control Your Drinking*. The basic components of our model include the following: (1) deciding what one wants from drinking; (2) setting limits; (3) counting drinks and monitoring drinking behavior; (4) altering how and what one drinks; and (5) managing the drinking situation. These particular foci were developed on the basis of the ways college students drink, the developmental and environmental factors that have a strong influence on students' drinking behavior, and our clinical observations over more than a decade in working with high-risk college drinkers. Through the provision of advice, we ultimately want to encourage students to reevaluate their patterns of drinking and to develop plans for lower-risk drinking.

Before moving to the specifics of each of these components, we again want to make several comments about process. The clinical basics for moderation training, as for any other form of advice giving, are as follows:

1. The therapist needs to meet the student **where he or she is** with respect to readiness and interest to change.

2. The therapist should avoid "pushing" a student into something he or she is not yet ready for. An artful balance needs to be maintained between accepting where the student is and "pulling" the student in the direction of change. "Pushing," like being shoved, involves moving a person to a place against his or her will, and can result in psychological reactance. In contrast to pushing, "pulling" in this context implies using clinical strategies and wisdom to help move the student in the direction of change.

3. The therapist should negotiate with the student about what to try. Once the negotiation is complete, the therapist should seek a verbal commitment from the student to do it.

Deciding What One Wants from Drinking. Seldom do students figure out how much they intend to drink on a particular occasion or how they intend to stop drinking. When asked how they decide how much to drink and when to stop, many students admit that they have never really considered the question before. Some will say that they will quit "right before I am about ready to throw up." Others admit that they don't quit "until the beer runs out"—obviously a risky plan, in light of the prevalence of kegs at many college and university parties. Such comments tend to emphasize that drinking behavior for many college students is under the control of external or environmental factors (e.g., the availability of alcoholic beverages), or is limited only by physical loss of control (e.g., passing out, throwing up, etc.).

The first bit of advice is to encourage students to critically consider what they want from drinking, as well as ways to drink that assure that they will achieve the fun they desire and get what they want while minimizing their risks from drinking. In keeping with our attempts to enhance motivation to change behavior, students ultimately need to realize on their own that what they stand to gain through moderate drinking far surpasses what they stand to lose. The therapist's role may be to facilitate a process by which the student can see that the benefits outweigh the losses. We have found that the more explicit and concrete the therapist can make the examples, the better. Just as a therapist can perform a mathematical calculation of potential monetary savings from reducing the student's tolerance to alcohol (see Dialogue 5.5, above), the therapist can provide specific examples of the actual calories in a favored beverage for students concerned about their weight (e.g., a can of beer contains the same number of calories as a hot dog or candy bar). Table 5.3 lists various negative consequences that can be avoided and positive consequences that can be gained through moderation; other items can be added in both columns, depending on the particular student.

TABLE 5.3. What a Student Can Avoid and Gain through Moderation

What a student can avoid	What a student can gain
Hangovers	Greater pleasure from lower BAL
Embarrassment	Financial savings
Weight gain	Improved scholastic performance
Pressure from family/school about grades	Greater control
Long-term health consequences	Others?
Tolerance and a heavy drinking pattern	
Others?	

Another method for eliciting this information from the student is to have him or her evaluate the short- and long-term pros and cons, as illustrated in Table 5.4. Although it is unlikely that there will be adequate time during the second session for the student to complete such an evaluation, making use of this table conceptually can be very helpful. The therapist might, for example, ask the student to broadly consider all reasons he or she can think of to change his or her current pattern of use and all reasons to maintain the status quo. It is important that the therapist balance this discussion by articulating both the pros and cons of changing and maintaining the status quo.

A word of caution: It is important here that the therapist listen to what the **student** wants from the experience, without inserting his or her own values or opinions about whether what the student wants is particularly important, worthy, or relevant. Although this seems on the surface of things to be a relatively simple matter, we have often found it difficult for therapists to listen accurately to what students are saying here. Because the success of this task hinges on eliciting reasons for change that are salient to a student, it is important for a therapist to pay careful, nonjudgmental attention.

Setting Limits. Once the student decides that the benefits of changing the drinking pattern outweigh maintaining the status quo, the second step is to assist the student in determining a drinking limit. Before this can be done, it is important for the student to learn a critical point that will aid him or her in defining what constitutes a **standard drink**: The student must pay attention to the particular amount of ethanol in a beverage, since all drinks vary in actual strength. Miller and Rollnick (1991) use the following convention for defining one drink: ½ ounce of pure ethanol. So what constitutes a drink? Some standardized drink equivalents have been provided in connection with use of the BDP in Chapter 4, but here is a more detailed list:

- 1 ounce of 100 proof distilled spirits

- 1¼ ounces of 80-proof distilled spirits

- 2½ ounces of fortified wine (sherry, port, etc.) @ 20% alcohol

• • •

TABLE 5.4. Pros and Cons of Moderating Alcohol Use

Short term		Long term	
Pros	Cons	Pros	Cons
Moderating alcohol use			
• Can remain in control. • Less risky. • Fewer hangovers or side effects. • Cheaper. • Don't have to worry about being a jerk or offending people.	• May sacrifice some fun. • Will have to pay attention to how much alcohol is consumed. • Interruption of spontaneity.	• Maintain good health. • Have chance of doing better in school, which will improve chances for job/graduate school. • Enjoy positive social reputation.	• Might sacrifice some friends who drink more heavily. • Might forgo some activities that could have been fun.
Maintaining status quo			
• Having fun with friends. • Fitting in. • "Cutting loose." • Way to celebrate. • Doing risky things can be fun.	• Social embarrassment. • Involvement in risky behaviors (e.g., getting in accident while driving).	• Really live it up during college before "reality" sets in. • More money spent.	• Less successful in school than could have been.

• 4 ounces of table wine @ 12% alcohol

• 10 ounces of wine cooler @ 5% alcohol

• 10 ounces of beer @ 5% alcohol

• 12 ounces of beer @ 4% alcohol

Because the goal of moderation training is avoidance of problematic or harmful use of alcohol, several different drinking goals can be set: (1) the maximum number of drinks consumed per day; (2) the maximum number of drinks consumed per week; and (3) the maximum approximate BAL achieved at all times (Hester, 1995). Specific advice about drinking limits should be tailored to the individual's stage of change—that is, his or her interest in and readiness for change. Because many of the heavy-drinking students we meet with are in the precontemplation stage, we tend to advise taking only one reasonably simple step toward setting limits on their drinking. Students who are more eager to modify their use may instead be asked to consider setting all three kinds of limit goals.

We typically begin a discussion of limit setting by asking the following question: "How do you decide how much to drink?" After eliciting implicit strategies, we then suggest alternative methods. For some students, it may be simplest to have an across-the-board rule about the maximum number of drinks they allow themselves per occasion.

Because negative health consequences increase dramatically when more than three drinks per day are consumed (Klatsky & Armstrong, 1993; Klatsky, Friedman, & Giegelaub, 1981; Saunders & Aasland, 1987), Hester (1995) recommends that clients do not exceed three drinks per day, and further advises against daily drinking. The NIAAA (1992) has recommended a maximum limit of two drinks per day for men, and one drink per day for women. However, a limit of 3 drinks per day for a precontemplative college drinker accustomed to 10–15 drinks may not be realistic or "do-able." Balancing health and safety concerns and standards with pragmatism, the therapist will need to collaborate with the student in arriving at what seems like a reasonable daily limit, if this is the direction pursued. Here it is important to keep a principal tenet of harm reduction in mind: Any movement in the direction of reduction of risks or harm is better than no movement at all.

When possible, we prefer that students set their drinking limits by using a BAL standard, since the majority of alcohol-related problems occur under conditions of excessive intoxication. Any increased commitment and effort to reduce the degree of intoxication will probably result in a concomitant reduction in problems. Furthermore, committing to a BAL limit is often a smaller step in the right direction than asking a student not to exceed a quantity total in many cases. We generally recommend a limit of 0.05% or 0.06% BAL because a nontolerant person is likely to experience a mild buzz but is unlikely to become intoxicated at such a limit. This may not be realistic or desirable for the unconcerned heavy drinker with a moderate degree of tolerance to alcohol. The therapist can introduce the idea of setting a BAL limit as follows:

> "There are a lot of ways adults figure out how to moderate their drinking. Some people simply decide a maximum number of drinks they can drink per day. Others come up with a weekly limit. Still others concentrate more on the ceiling of how 'buzzed' they get, which is usually based on an estimate of their BAL. In some cases, the person might do all of the above. In your case, I would recommend that you consider setting a BAL that is within a safe range while still enabling you to get what you want from alcohol. Often the best way to do this is by experimenting with different BALS and determining your point of diminishing return."

In setting a BAL limit, a student may decide first to reduce his or her tolerance to alcohol, and then to set a "reasonable limit" such as 0.05%. Another student may decide to reduce the BAL limit incrementally over time (e.g., by using behavioral principles of shaping). We minimally recommend that students experiment with finding the "right" limit for them by doing the following:

- Exploring the effects of alcohol at lower BALs.

- Establishing a **point of diminishing return**—that is, a point at which one more drink produces no additional stimulating effects, but instead increases the depressant effects from alcohol (the biphasic response).

- Maximizing what they like and minimizing what they don't like.

Occasionally, students will choose a BAL limit that poses health risks or problems; we typically consider such a limit as being 0.08% or greater. When this occurs, it is usually because a student has difficulty envisioning still being able to have fun while drinking less, particularly when his or her peers are intoxicated. In these situations, it is important for the therapist to understand these concerns in a supportive fashion, while remaining appropriately concerned about the student's well-being.

What direction the therapist chooses to take at this point depends to a large extent on the rapport between the student and therapist, the student's perception of risk and degree of readiness, and how far the therapist feels he or she can go before creating additional reactance. Although the situation will vary from case to case, we believe it is important for the therapist to continue to exhibit an appropriate level of concern, but to respect the student's ultimate decision. It is our hope that resistant students who have a positive experience during the brief intervention will be more likely to consider the contact from the interview upon leaving or to request services from us or someone else in the future.

On occasion, a student may express no interest in moderating alcohol use in certain high-risk settings. In these situations, we recommend that the therapist ask the student about his or her alcohol outcome expectancies (e.g., feeling uninhibited) and the BAL "required" to get the effect. The therapist can also ask whether there are any effects the student wishes to avoid (e.g., vomiting, hangovers). The therapist can then suggest that the student work toward a balanced drinking style that will help him or her avoid the negative effects while still getting experiencing the pleasurable effects. We hypothesize that students are more likely to experiment with this common-sense strategy if they leave the session with a clear, concrete direction.

Knowing how to refuse drinks is an important part of setting (and maintaining) limits. Most students can generate a number of drink refusal statements when prompted during the session. The real question is whether they can apply this skill in the real context of their lives when it's needed. We encourage students to start honing their drink refusal skills by overlearning these skills through practice. It's sometimes helpful to have a few overlearned, patterned responses that require little thought to generate in a party context. Listed below are some examples:

- "No, thanks."

- "No, thanks. I'm going to wait a bit."

- "No, thanks. I've reached my limit for the night."

- "I have to get up early tomorrow. No, thanks."

Many students have already refused drinks at one time or another. If time permits, we ask how they did it and how well it went. Students are often concerned about negative evaluation by peers if they refuse a drink. **We encourage students to practice refusing**

drinks just for the sake of building their skills, so that they will have them when they want/need them.

Counting Drinks and Monitoring Drinking Behavior. The next step is to count drinks when drinking. Ideally, students wishing to moderate their use of alcohol will continue to complete monitoring cards for a month or so, identifying occasions when they are either tempted to exceed or do exceed the limit, in order to prepare better for future high-risk occasions. We ourselves have rarely made this recommendation to students, and generally only in cases where motivation to moderate drinking is very high and commitment is strong. More typically, we focus on simple strategies students can use in the moment to keep track of their drinks. The general rule, as is the case with all interventions that focus on building motivation to change, is for therapists to take what they can get and get what they can take in the way of commitment to action. As always, the trick is to be flexible, creative, realistic, and nonjudgmental, remembering that any amount of monitoring is better than no monitoring at all and that monitoring a behavior can by itself change the behavior.

The list below provides some suggestions for how a student might monitor his or her drinking:

• Prior to a party or drinking occasion, the student figures out the maximum number of drinks to be consumed (on the basis of a total count or BAL calculation). The student places this many coins in one pocket, each one representing one drink. As the student starts to consume a new drink, he or she moves one coin into an empty pocket.

• The student uses a golf-clicker to count each drink. Golf-clickers are small in size and easily palmed in one's hand or placed in one's pocket.

• Prior to having each drink, the student takes a moment to remember the number of drinks already consumed.

• The student brings exactly the number of drinks he or she intends to consume to a party, and creates a rule that he or she will drink **only** these beverages. A variation of this is for the student to bring his or her own minus the number of drinks the student intends to borrow or share with others, or the number the student plans to consume plus the number he or she typically gives to or shares with others.

Altering How and What One Drinks. The best way to determine what to alter in order to reduce the risks associated with drinking—that is, how to "tweak" the situational factors associated with high-risk situations—is to review the monitoring cards or the episodic portion of the BDP for factors associated with risky drinking. In one case, a student consistently drank to intoxication when he was with friends from high school and they were consuming his favorite drink, a certain brand of whiskey. It was only within this specific context that his drinking became, from his perspective, out of control. He was anticipating attending a high school friend's wedding in a month and expressed concern about overdrinking, because he knew that there would be many occasions to party with his buddies and drink whiskey. He decided to "tweak" the situational factors in the service of his moderation goals by not drinking whiskey and instead drinking microbrewed beers, which he would bring with him to the parties. As this example illustrates, the best plan to alter how a student drinks is one that is personalized to the student's interests in combination with his or her specific situational cues.

A number of different strategies will allow a student to control his or her drinking rate in a way that does not compromise fun or enjoyment. Listed below are some generic strategies that are generally useful in efforts to moderate use.

- *Switching from more potent beverages with higher ethanol concentrations or percentages to weaker or lighter beverages.* This might include selecting beer over hard alcohol, or a light beer over an ale.

- *Slowing down the pace of drinking.* College students in particular tend to gulp drinks, either as a drinking style or in the context of drinking games; as a subfeature of this tactic, we recommend that students avoid drinking games. Hester (1995) recommends a sipping rate of 60 seconds. Although this rate offers a standard, the therapist should be ready to negotiate a rate that is satisfactory to the student and represents a slowing of the existing rates. Another strategy is to set an overall rate for consuming the total drink. For example, the student might set a rule that he or she will take 45 minutes to consume each beverage.

- *Spacing drinks further apart.* Just as a student can set a time rule for how long he or she will take to consume a drink, the student can also set a time rule with respect to the period of time that elapses between one drink and the next. A related strategy is to determine the amount of time that will need to pass between drinks by dividing the total number of drinks to be consumed by the lengths of time the student plans to drink.

- *Alternating nonalcoholic beverages with alcoholic beverages.* Students often indicate that they feel somewhat awkward drinking nonalcoholic beverages when partying with friends. This appears to be especially true for younger students looking to "fit in" with older students, or for students who do not know their drinking peers particularly well (e.g., those who have just moved to a new floor of a residence hall, who are drinking with other new members of their sorority or fraternity pledge class, etc.) There are several ways around this obstacle. For example, a student can drink a nonalcoholic beverage from a paper cup so as to disguise the contents, or he or she might choose a drink that looks like an alcoholic beverage but is actually alcohol-free (e.g., nonalcoholic beer). For students unwilling to do this or make other compromises, the principles of harm reduction direct the therapist to suggest other risk-reducing alternatives, such as alternating potent drinks with less potent drinks.

Managing the Drinking Situation. Managing one's own drinking situation involves taking a more complex and reflexive analysis of drinking. It requires a constant process of stepping back and examining what works, what isn't working, and what factors (e.g., barriers, other situational factors, etc.) are getting in the way of pursuing moderate drinking. On occasion, this might also include identifying and seeking out functional alternatives to drinking (e.g., exercise, relaxation, etc.). Once the additional factors are identified, the individual can begin problem-solving solutions to these newly identified factors and tinkering with the plan in a trial-and-error fashion.

Offering a Prospective Outlook: Preparing the Road Ahead

In cases where students' risks for problems are high but their concern is low, we focus on preparing the students for possible problems that could lie ahead and on enabling them to recognize specific problems in themselves or their friends. We suggest that a therapist simply ask such a student "How might you recognize if you are having a problem with alcohol in the future?" The more specific behaviors the student and therapist can generate, the better. Students often describe a series of potentially problematic negative consequences from drinking or extreme behaviors (e.g., "I would pass out or have blackouts every time I drank," "My grades would fall"; "I might get arrested for drunk driving"). Although this is a step in the right direction, the next step is to help the student identify earlier events in the chain leading up to these kinds of problems (e.g., "I would miss a lot of classes from being hung over," "I would turn in my assignments late," "I would drive a lot after I had been drinking heavily"). We also suggest that the therapist encourage the student to consider a less risky frame of reference to determine whether there's a problem:

> "The behaviors you mentioned are often ones that develop after drinking in a very risky way for some time. By the time you get to this point, the negative consequences are pretty unpleasant and substantial. I wonder what kinds of behaviors you might notice earlier on, before things reached this level."

Addressing General Lifestyle Behaviors

The importance of giving advice and making recommendations about general lifestyle behaviors should not be gauged by the limited amount of space devoted to it here. Future research may find that one of the most effective ways to modify drinking behavior is to create functional alternatives to drinking alcohol (e.g., meditation, golf, virtual reality "escapes," etc.). Indeed, many of our research participants commented in their closing interviews that if they had other options for socializing with peers on the weekends in a semistructured, enjoyable way, they would opt for these activities. Some recommended that residence halls take more initiative in planning floor or dorm events away from the dorm or campus. The key to success, they reported, would lie in the ability of the staff to figure out the events their residents would actually attend.

New lifestyle behaviors can either serve as structural alternatives to drinking, as described above (e.g., going on a night hike can be an alternative to going to a party), or can reduce the motivation to drink. Changing a student's motivation to drink (and ultimately the actual drinking behavior) can occur through an indirect, back-door process when a competing motivation, such as getting healthy or more centered is increased. It is not uncommon for people who begin exercising regularly to begin eating more healthily as well. An earlier study by Marlatt and colleagues found that students who began a practice of meditation or regular exercise also significantly reduced their use of alcohol. This approach, which focuses on the student's lifestyle goals (regardless of whether the goals involve drinking alcohol), may prove to be one of the most effective ways to reduce harmful effects from heavy drinking in college students.

Referral for Medical Consultation

When students present with signs of moderate to severe alcohol dependence, or with medical conditions in which alcohol use may be contraindicated, it is important to advise that the students consult a physician. On occasion, we will recommend that a student consult a physician about obtaining liver function tests to determine possible acute or chronic liver damage. Although this can enhance the student's motivation to quit or cut back on alcohol use if tests are positive, it can have the opposite impact if results are negative. For this reason, it may be more effective to recommend liver function tests only for those students with moderate to severe alcohol dependence.

Making Referrals

On occasion, we refer students for outside services. The most common referrals are to other mental health professionals for ongoing individual psychotherapy. Other referrals, although less frequent, are occasionally made to physicians for a medical consultation and liver function tests (see above), and to self-help groups such as Rational Recovery and Alcoholics Anonymous.

To smooth the way, we recommend contacting the campus mental health services center and the primary health care center well in advance of referring students to them, in order to establish the best routes for referral. We have also found it helpful to know the answers to commonly asked questions about these services, including the cost for services; special restrictions or exclusion criteria a clinic may have; whether a clinic has a waiting list, and if so, how long it is; and so on. Information about meetings of self-help groups on campus and in the university area should be made widely available.

The key to a successful referral outcome is preparing the student for the referral. We recommend the following guidelines for facilitating a referral to another mental health professional; these guidelines can be modified for use with other types of referrals.

1. The therapist should orient the student to the school's mental health services (e.g., screening procedures, initial intake, cost of services, etc., for each of the facilities available to students) and to services outside the campus community (when these are available).

2. If possible, the therapist should provide the student with a handout that describes the various agencies and provides information on how to contact them.

3. The therapist should explain that it typically takes time to find the "right" person to work with.

4. The student should be asked what kind of mental help professional he or she would prefer to work with; gender preference, stylistic preference (e.g., someone who listens mostly, who is more casual and "down to earth," who can give explicit advice, etc.), and other factors should be considered.

5. The therapist should coach the student on how to convey these preferences to the intake counselor and to the therapist he or she is eventually assigned.

6. When possible, the therapist should allow the student to make the initial contact from the place where the BASICS session is being held (this increases the probability that the student will follow through).

Taking the Next Step: Stepped Care

Students who have difficulty implementing moderation after BASICS, or who continue to drink in a hazardous or risky fashion, can be "bumped up" a notch to the next level of treatment intensity. We recommend that the ultimate choice of a treatment option be made by the student through a collaborative exchange with the therapist. Some stepped-care options we have offered are described below.

Follow-Up Booster BASICS Session(s)

An appointment can be made for a 30- to 50-minute follow-up booster session. The appointment should be set far enough in the future to give the student sufficient time to apply the skills learned in BASICS. We typically schedule these appointments between 1 and 3 months after BASICS. When it appears that a follow-up session will be scheduled, the therapist should spend several minutes at the close of BASICS setting several specific behavioral goals to attempt during the interim period; the follow-up session then begins with a review of the student's progress on these goals. The therapist next reinforces gains made, and spends the remainder of the booster session troubleshooting solutions to the barriers (if any) that have interfered with achieving the goals. The decision of whether to set a second follow-up session should be made by the student and therapist, based on the usefulness of the first. Upon terminating contact with the therapist, the student should be reminded that services remain available, should he or she need to consult with a therapist in the future.

Correspondence Course

For purposes of a previous research study comparing the effectiveness of several ASTP modalities (Kivlahan et al., 1990), a manual was written for the correspondence course treatment condition. The manual (described in Chapter 2) is structured as a workbook and guides the student through a series of lessons and exercises that capture the essential components of ASTP. Students most likely to benefit from the *Alcohol Skills Training Manual* are those who enjoy reading and are highly motivated to change. The manual can be used in conjunction with other options. Sections of the manual most pertinent to the student's needs and interests can also be assigned; the material can then be discussed in later booster sessions or in subsequent telephone contacts.

Behavior Change Course for Credit

We offer a two-credit course in self-directed behavioral change through the Department of Psychology at the University of Washington. While learning about the theory and research related to behavior change, students experientially apply the course knowledge to altering a targeted behavior. *Self-Directed Behavior: Self-Modification for Personal Adjustment* (Watson & Tharp, 1993) is an excellent textbook for such a course and can be augmented with the *Alcohol Skills Training Manual* (see above) for students interested in modifying their drinking behavior.

Psychoeducational Short-Term or Long-Term Group

A brief psychoeducational group format can be used to introduce group participants to the ASTP curriculum. These groups can vary in length from two sessions (using BASICS in a group context) to six to eight sessions (using the *Alcohol Skills Training Manual* as a guidebook and/or textbook). For students in need of more intensive work or a more involved process, a process-oriented treatment approach focusing on issues involved in alcohol abuse and relapse prevention can be recommended (see Vannicelli, 1992).

Individual Counseling

Occasionally within the context of indicated prevention programming, use of alcohol may be found to be connected with a great deal of emotional distress, including adjustment difficulties, anxiety, or depression. Although this is certainly not always the case, these affective difficulties can result in increased use of alcohol and difficulty in moderating or abstaining from use. In such a situation, a student may benefit from a course of individual counseling or therapy. Within the context of prevention work, counseling should include relapse prevention strategies for behavior change and maintenance.

Referral to Moderation-Based Groups

Several new group programs are available for people who want to receive group support while pursuing a moderation goal. A new self-help group, Moderation Management, has recently been formed for people interested in moderating their use of alcohol. Founded by Audrey Kishline, Moderation Management offers participants social support in addition to specific skill-building strategies based on controlled-drinking treatment outcome studies. Persons interested in this program can learn more about it by reading Kishline's (1994) *Moderate Drinking: The New Option for Problem Drinkers.*

DrinkWise, a moderation program developed by researchers at the University of Michigan offers several cognitive-behavioral treatment routes to choose from: individual, group, or telephone counseling. The content of all three approaches is generally similar. Information about the DrinkWise program can be obtained through the Health Promotions Division of the University of Michigan Medical Center or through their web site (http://wwwmed.umich.edu/drinkwise).

Referral to Abstinence-Based Self-Help Groups

Students who manifest signs of alcohol dependence, and who are self-identified "alcoholics" or "problem drinkers" who want to quit drinking altogether, may benefit from participation in an abstinence-based self-help group such as Alcoholics Anonymous or Rational Recovery. Although these two groups share a view that abstinence is the goal for life, they differ widely in their understanding of addiction problems and their approach to sobriety.

Alcoholics Anonymous views alcohol problems as stemming from spiritual alienation from a Higher Power (Nowinski, Baker, & Carroll, 1994). Although there is some recognition that alcohol problems stem to some extent from a physiological disease process comparable to an allergy, the essence of the process of recovery lies in the Twelve Steps and Twelve Traditions. Emergence from the addictive process is accomplished once the person admits powerlessness over alcohol and turns his or her life over to the "care of God as we understand Him." The focus in Alcoholics Anonymous on a Higher Power is a draw for many newcomers, but a distancer for others. Though many atheists and agnostics are comfortable with tailoring the program to their needs (e.g., focusing on the group as the Higher Power, instead of a classic Christian God figure), many have found this perceived focus on religion intolerable or counterproductive.

Rational Recovery is based on Albert Ellis's rational– emotive therapy and places the locus of control for change in the hands of the individual with support from the group (rather than in a Higher Power, as in Alcoholics Anonymous). Alcoholics learn ways to cope with the urges and cravings that disrupt their consciousness as they attempt abstinence. Rather than making a commitment for life to "recovering" by attending meetings, sponsoring newcomers, and carrying the message to other alcoholics throughout one's life (as suggested by Alcoholics Anonymous), Rational Recovery encourages firm participation and commitment for 6 months, after which time an abstinent addict is considered "recovered."

We recommend that students considering this type of self-help group decide for themselves which approach to choose. Students may be provided with a brief overview of how each program approaches recovering from addictions. It is advised that students explore several different meetings of both groups, to make sure they receive a fair representation of what each program has to offer.

Referral to Intensive Outpatient or Inpatient Hospitalization

For clients who are severely alcohol-dependent, who feel out of control, and who have had no success with other programming, referral to an abstinence-oriented recovery program is recommended.

CHAPTER 6

- •
- •
- •

Clinical Considerations

The objective of this chapter is to enable therapists to anticipate and respond to common clinical concerns and pitfalls encountered when implementing BASICS. Included in this review are a theoretical and practical discussion of integrating motivational interviewing and skills training; a typology of common student responses to the brief intervention and strategies for working with each of these common responses; and ways of troubleshooting responses to other common clinical situations.

Suggestions for Integrating Motivational Interviewing and Skills Training

Types of Student Responses to BASICS

Categorizing Common Student Responses
The Determined Student
The Precontemplative and Open Student
The Precontemplative and Defensive Student
The Maintenance Student

Troubleshooting Sticky Situations

Working with "Bravado" Drinkers
Working with Sanctioned Students
Reactant Abstinence

SUGGESTIONS FOR INTEGRATING MOTIVATIONAL INTERVIEWING AND SKILLS TRAINING

The most common problem in BASICS arises when a therapist attempts to do skills training before sufficient motivation is cultivated in a student. For example, precontemplative students who are at considerable risk for negative consequences of drinking but express little concern about their drinking are seldom interested in setting limits or discussing ways to say "no." **In these circumstances, the skills training portion of**

BASICS must be minimized and motivational enhancement efforts must be maximized. Getting a commitment to try out moderate drinking may occur quickly, leaving plenty of time for skills training. Until motivation is enhanced and a commitment is achieved, however, teaching such students moderation strategies will constitute "putting the cart before the horse."

Discord also commonly arises when the advice and information provided are not commensurate to the student's level of readiness. Again, this occurs most often with precontemplative students who express little concern about their drinking, but who are nonetheless at considerable risk for alcohol-related problems. In these instances, therapists may find themselves ambushing the students with advice, hoping that something will eventually sink in through a "sleeper" effect. More often than not, students react to the deluge with increased reactance, as manifested by indifference, boredom, and passivity during the interview.

One effective way to avoid this trap is to sidestep it by assuming a nonjudgmental, non-problem-focused tone and clarifying the main objective of BASICS early in the interview process. One way to do this is to normalize the need for feedback:

> "As you may know, it is quite common for students' drinking patterns to change significantly when they enter college from high school. It has been our experience that students are seldom taught how to drink alcohol in a safe way; in this respect, learning to drink is like learning how to drive, how to use power tools, or how to do other potentially risky things. The purpose of this session is for us to look at your drinking pattern, identify any possible risks associated with your use of alcohol, and come up with some strategies you can use in the future to minimize these risks while still having fun. What you ultimately do with this information, however, is entirely up to you."

Another strategy to avoid reactance is to provide feedback, information, and advice in a fashion that gives the student a choice about how to receive the content. Rollnick, Heather, and Bell (1992) advise therapists to "choose the right moment and ask for permission," preferably when clients seem curious or ask for the information. In a neutral fashion, a therapist might ask, "I wonder whether you would be interested in knowing more about [topic]." Of course, the therapist must be accepting of a negative response. In addition to using a neutral, nonjudgmental tone, the therapist can also provide the student with the opportunity to process the information, particularly when the student is interested in or alarmed by the presented material. For example, the therapist might ask a reflective question ("What do you make of all this?") or amplify the student's visible concerns ("You seem quite surprised by that information").

In summary, motivational interviewing and skills training arise from different but complementary theoretical and practical perspectives. We believe that integration of the two is not only possible but beneficial, particularly in working with college students. The simplest integration is matching the proportion of these two approaches to a student's level of readiness. For precontemplative and contemplative students, motivational interviewing is more heavily weighed; for those who are ready to make changes, skills training can be emphasized. A more complex and perhaps difficult integration is to realize that good skills training must take motivation into account. A therapist should suggest skill-building exercises that not only are appropriate to motivational level, but also serve to increase motivation. For example, self-monitoring (perhaps the most commonly used behavioral task), when presented as a technique for the student and therapist to "learn more" about the behavior in question, usually serves to enhance the student's motivation to change the behavior. Motivational interviewing can also be used as a frame not only for providing personal feedback, but also for (softly) confronting commonly held beliefs about alcohol effects and social norms, for discussing common approaches to changing behavior, and for setting goals for change. Creating a nonjudgmental tone, allowing the student to choose, and providing processing time are all strategies that facilitate consideration of change, and hence greater motivation and use of skills.

TYPES OF STUDENT RESPONSES TO BASICS

It would certainly be nice if each student, regardless of his or her position on the stages-of-change continuum prior to BASICS, could successfully conclude the brief intervention with a plan in hand. Unfortunately, this is neither a realistic nor a healthy expectation to hold, as it can only lead a therapist to feel that he or she has failed or done something wrong if action does not immediately follow BASICS. This section introduces the reader to the most common student responses to BASICS, and describes clinical approaches to these different response styles.

Categorizing Common Student Responses

We have found it useful to categorize student responses to BASICS along two dimensions: (1) a student's current degree of risk for alcohol-related problems or hazardous behaviors, and (2) the student's expressed degree of interest in changing his or her drinking behavior. Figure 6.1 illustrates these conditions across the two dimensions. Because we target high-risk drinkers for indicated preventive intervention in BASICS, we only occasionally encounter students with a low degree of risk who are nonetheless highly concerned about their drinking pattern (the **"worried well"**). More commonly, students receiving BASICS fall into one of the other three categories upon entering the intervention: high risk with commensurate concern and interest in changing behavior (**determined**); low current risk with prior history of higher risk and current low degree of concern (**maintenance**); and high risk but low degree of concern or interest in change (**precontemplative**). The precontemplative group can be further subdivided into two subcategories (**receptive** and **defensive**), based on students' degree of openness or resistance as the interview progresses.

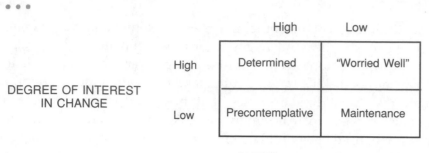

FIGURE 6.1. Typology of student responses to BASICS.

The Determined Student

Along with the precontemplative, receptive student, the determined student is often the easiest and most gratifying type to work with. Such a student is at considerable risk and is generally ready to make use of whatever resources he or she receives. The working alliance between therapist and student tends to develop with relative ease early in the session and to build throughout. These students often appear engaged by the purpose and content of the interview, are alarmed by their severity of risk, and are forthcoming with ideas and information that may be helpful in moving into an action phase. These students will in effect say, "I had no idea it was this bad. Wow. I've got to do something about this."

Because the determined student's motivation to change is high, greater amounts of session time can be devoted to developing a specific risk-reducing plan and to experimenting with new behavioral approaches, such as practicing drink refusal in an imagined high-risk setting. The specific tasks of the therapist are to assist the student in mapping out an action plan that is realistic and attainable.

The Precontemplative and Receptive Student

The precontemplative and receptive student also presents with a high degree of risk, but has given little thought to his or her drinking prior to receiving BASICS. Typically, such students react with surprise and disbelief upon receiving normative feedback. They often comment, "Are you sure? That can't be right. The people you studied probably didn't respond honestly, so they looked good." However, as the feedback continues and rapport builds during the session, the skepticism is replaced by outward signs of concern and perturbed comments (e.g., "Wow. I can't believe this. It's kind of scary").

To increase this receptiveness still further, it is important for the therapist to reflect the student's reactions and concern (e.g., "You seemed quite surprised; you really didn't expect to find such a difference between your pattern and most of your peers," or

"What's it like for you to receive this feedback?"), and then to continue with the feedback. The interview should conclude by setting concrete goals commensurate to the student's readiness for change and skills enhancement. When students are not ready to make specific plans, general goals (e.g., "I am going to consider this") are quite acceptable.

Consider the case of a 19-year-old female student living in a university residence hall. Prior to the second BASICS session, Sherry was unconcerned by her use of alcohol and considered herself a light drinker in contrast to many of her friends. Typically, Sherry consumed approximately eight beers on each of three occasions per week, placing her in the 95th percentile when her quantity of drinking was compared to that of other college students. In addition, Sherry commonly obtained very elevated BALs when she drank (0.16%), and on occasion obtained even higher BALs (monthly peak was estimated at 0.25%). Although Sherry had experienced some negative effects (e.g., occasional hangovers and embarrassing occasions), she had fortunately experienced few serious negative consequences from her heavy drinking. During the initial interview, Sherry stated that she was raised in a small rural town, where "partying in someone's barn" on weekend nights was the most common social activity among her high school classmates.

Sherry expressed alarm early in the feedback session after receiving her percentile ranking and BAL scores, commenting, "I can't believe it. I had no idea." Extending the student's concern further, the therapist gently focused on eliciting Sherry's feelings and reactions to this feedback. Because Sherry had mentioned earlier that much of her drinking occurred with her male friends, the therapist compared Sherry's BAL for a typical drinking occasion to the level obtained by a male counterpart (based on an estimate of his weight). Sherry again reacted with surprise and concern; she had not previously considered the differences in weight and alcohol metabolism for men and women. Sherry's interest and concern provided the opportunity for the therapist to weave in information about important gender differences, while also allowing Sherry to examine her reactions to this content. Within a brief period of time, Sherry had moved from precontemplation to contemplation and seemed headed into action. In order to build Sherry's interest in change still further, the therapist proceeded with the session, providing feedback about risks and information about alcohol.

Since the remaining content of the session served to strengthen Sherry's interest in changing her drinking patterns, the therapist devoted the last 10 minutes of the session to wrapping things up. The therapist commented, "You've been given a lot of information today that seemed new and surprising. I commend you for listening so openly to the information and asking such good questions. I noticed at times that it was a little difficult at times to do so, but you persisted anyway. I respect that."

Because it was already clear that Sherry was interested in reducing her drinking habit, the therapist preceded to elicit a course of action from her while encouraging and reinforcing her decision to take action: "So, in light of our discussion today, what are you considering as the next step, if any?" Not surprisingly, Sherry was particularly concerned about her high BALs and the quantity of alcohol she consumed weekly, and wished to reduce both. The therapist commended her again on deciding to choose these as the goals, then inquired how Sherry wished to achieve these goals. Carefully modulating the amount of advice to provide, given Sherry's level of interest, the therapist provided a menu of suggestions or "tips" that she might consider in deciding how to proceed with her goals (e.g., setting a drinking/BAL goal in advance, then counting drinks; spacing drinks throughout the night; experimenting with not drinking; etc.).

Once the specific plan was set, the therapist then proceeded to inquire about possible barriers or roadblocks that might compromise it. In this fashion, any barriers could be anticipated and planned for. Sherry expressed vague concern that once she was in a drinking situation, she would have more difficulty than she could anticipate during the session. The therapist queried further to determine what might help Sherry overcome this obstacle, in light of Sherry's concerns. After a moment of problem-solving discussion, the therapist recommended that they set a meeting time in a few months to "check in," which was well received by Sherry. The therapist ultimately met with Sherry for two additional booster sessions. At the conclusion of the second of these sessions, Sherry felt that she would be able to continue to maintain the gains she had made on her own.

The Precontemplative and Defensive Student

We generally find sessions with precontemplative and defensive students the most challenging, as our concern for the students' health and well-being increases in an inverse relationship to their apparent lack of concern about risks. It is not uncommon for these students to state, "I'm really not concerned about this. This is just a part of my lifestyle for now," or "I don't see this as a problem. I would know it if I had a problem. This is just what my friends and I do together."

As noted earlier, in response to these students' apparent lack of interest, it is not uncommon for therapists to lecture the students in an attempt to ignite their concern or to incite a "sleeper" effect (i.e., to say something that will increase motivation several days, weeks, or months after the intervention). Unfortunately, we know of no empirical data that support delayed onset of the therapeutic value of the intervention. For this reason, we believe it is more beneficial in the long run to focus on motivational enhancement within the context of the sessions in these cases. Efforts aimed at increasing a precontemplative clients' perception of risks and problems associated with his or her drinking are preferred over the dissemination of information and advice.

Another common mistake made by therapists in these situations is to move into the action phase before the students are ready to do so. Although learning alternatives to heavy drinking sometimes enhances motivation to change, leaping too far into a program of change before a student is ready (e.g., providing tips on ways to reduce alcohol consumption) can trigger psychological reactance instead of facilitating change. With a precontemplative and defensive student, it is especially important for the therapist to present both skills and information that are commensurate with the degree of motivation. Again, a better approach may be to focus on exploring the motivational factors that reinforce heavy drinking, as well as the short-term and long-term costs and benefits of maintaining the status quo versus changing current behavior.

For purposes of illustration, Nick, an 18-year-old freshman living in a university residence hall, was among our high-risk sample of volunteers to receive BASICS. He presented during the initial session as a warm, intelligent young man with a pleasant sense of humor. He interacted openly with the therapist and was interested in exchanging ideas about alcohol use among college students. He told of a high school friend who was killed during a spring recess in a vehicular accident while intoxicated. The death of his friend had upset him and his close network of friends greatly, and caused them to reflect on their own drinking behavior. Nick described his "successful" efforts to moderate his drinking since this event.

Despite the stated magnitude of his loss and his decision to cut down on his alcohol use in an effort to reduce his risks, Nick described consuming approximately 80 drinks on average per week, typically reaching a BAL of about 0.25%. Although Nick did not mention any negative consequences of his alcohol use during the initial interview, his endorsement of RAPI items on the paper-and-pencil questionnaires suggested to the therapist that he was experiencing a number of such consequences. An analysis of the information gained from the initial interview revealed a young man at enormous risk for multiple kinds of alcohol-related problems who instead perceived himself at little risk, having mastered potential risks "successfully" in the past.

Within many treatment programs, this discrepancy between Nick's risk and his perception of risk—or, stated another way, his unwillingness or inability to comprehend the enormity of his risk—would possibly be viewed as a symptom of denial. Although Nick may indeed have been denying the severity of his alcohol abuse and related risk, we believe that it is functionally more useful in a case like his to sidestep the issue of denial entirely. Instead, the therapist focused the second session on facilitating Nick's movement from precontemplation to contemplation. Following the protocol for the second session, the therapist reviewed the individualized feedback with Nick. He received the information in a seemingly open fashion, continuing, however, to discount the risks being described. Though he did not say so directly, Eric's comments about the feedback implied the following: He felt confident that he was not at risk for alcohol problems; he could cut back on his use if he so desired; he believed he would be able to recognize the warning signals if his alcohol use was becoming problematic; drinking heavily with his friends was a very pleasurable and desirable activity; and for all these reasons, he felt that there was really no reason to modify his pattern of drinking.

Following the review of individualized feedback, the therapist pursued two courses with Nick. First, she performed a cost–benefit analyses with him, inquiring about what he stood to gain and lose both in the short run and in the long run by maintaining his current drinking behavior versus reducing his use to moderate levels. Nick expressed that he felt he had much more to lose by changing his habits now, and more to gain if he moderated his use upon graduation. During this discussion, Nick mentioned the discomfort he imagined he would feel at being with his friends (many of whom he knows intimately from high school) and not joining in their drinking. He also mentioned his regret that he was unable to "get away" more from school because he had so little money for travel and other expenses. In a careful manner, so as not to ignite reactance, the therapist asked Nick whether he had considered buying less alcohol than usual for a period, in order to save for a particular trip. (By proceeding in this way with a client like Nick, a therapist reintroduces moderation goals within a frame that may make some pragmatic sense to the client. Should the client be interested, the door is then open for a discussion of specific moderation strategies. Furthermore, the client can experiment with these strategies without explicitly acknowledging risks or making a specific commitment to changing behavior, and can have the direct experience that drinking less does not necessarily result in having less fun.) Nick was interested in considering this as an option and seemed to have some ideas of how he might proceed. In light of his ambivalence, the therapist made no additional attempt to provide advice or strategies.

The second strategy pursued by the therapist was to explore with Nick how he could recognize whether he or someone close to him did have a problem with drinking in the future. The therapist had hoped to have Nick wrestle indirectly with what problem drinking might look like. Not surprisingly, Nick described an image of an individual with fairly substantial problems resulting from alcohol. Consistent with his self-assured sense of himself, he stated, "I would just know." The therapist persisted, encouraging Nick to describe the specific behaviors he would notice. When Nick's description continued to reflect behaviors consistent with severe alcohol problems, the therapist asked, "I wonder what you might notice a little earlier that might signal to you that trouble is around the corner—as a means of warning the person before the problems become so severe."

Although this case was unusual because of the degree of superficial openness displayed by Nick, it nonetheless illustrates the resistant style of a student who perceives his or her risk as low, despite a plethora of feedback to the contrary. Furthermore, it demonstrates the prioritizing of motivational enhancement within the precontemplative stage. The success of this approach is captured by Nick's written remarks, made following the second session on a program evaluation:

"The interview was very well done, and I thought the information was useful. Rather than an evangelistic-type sermon on the 'evils' of alcohol, the interviewer was logical, understanding, and warm. Only a logical discussion of drugs and drug use results in a logical thinking about drugs and usage by the interviewed."

The Maintenance Student

In the context of our Lifestyles research, students were targeted as "high-risk" on the basis of their personal risk factors during the spring semester of their senior year of high school. In many cases, 6 to 9 months had passed by the time these students received BASICS, and some had already significantly decreased their consumption of alcohol. Many attributed the change in their drinking behavior to maturational factors (e.g., increased academic demands and a desire to achieve scholastically, or "outgrowing" heavy partying). These students generally presented with low risks for future alcohol problems, due in part to their current low levels of consumption and their commitment to maintaining their current patterns. These students commonly remarked, "Yeah, I used to get pretty toasted, but I'm through with that now." When both objective and perceived risks are low, students may initially present as uninterested in the interview, since the information seems irrelevant to them. Indeed, a therapist confronted with such a student nay begin thinking, "This student doesn't need my help. He [she] is doing just fine."

Whereas it is important not to "push" a precontemplative student, providing only the basic tips for decreasing alcohol consumption to a maintenance student can result in a similar unfavorable outcome, as the student becomes increasingly irritated and bored with the interview process. A more appropriate approach to the second BASICS session with this student is to focus on maintenance strategies that will continue to facilitate low-risk behaviors. In doing so, it is important that the therapist reinforce the student's behavior by acknowledging his or her capability and by soliciting from the student maintenance-related topics to discuss during the second session. The discussion can take the form of brainstorming to generate additional skillful responses to the student's high-risk situations, or (better yet) ways the student can have even more fun while socializing with peers in ways that do not require (more) drinking.

To illustrate this point, consider the following recent interview with Tony, a 23-year-old fifth-year senior. Tony indicated that although he had once been a heavy drinker along with his fraternity brothers, for the past 2 years his drinking had gradually declined. At the time of the interview, his typical drinking pattern indicated that he drank significantly less than the average student norm, and he was unable to recall the last occasion he drank excessively. Early in the session, Tony presented as passive and uninterested, as he politely but indifferently responded to questions. He described feeling generally comfortable with setting limits and refusing drinks, and therefore did not feel the need for additional prevention "tips." The therapist then directed the session toward exploring potential high-risk episodic situations by asking, "If there were occasions when you might be tempted to drink heavily, what would they be?" Tony suddenly became engaged in conversation and described several high-risk situations in the near future, including his graduation and several upcoming bachelor parties.

Situational factors that might contribute to Tony's desire to drink excessively in these contexts were then explored. These high-risk situations included drinking with other men who typically "pound their drinks," the cultural tradition of drinking heavily on such occasions, and the presence of his favorite alcoholic beverage at these parties. The therapist performed a cost–benefit analysis with Tony by asking him to describe both the positive and negative aspects of drinking heavily at these upcoming occasions. Despite desiring to "cut loose" with his old friends, he didn't want to "make a fool of myself or wake up to the porcelain god in the morning." The therapist seized the moment to resolve the situational ambivalence in favor of moderate drinking, then worked toward helping Tony reduce his drinking in these particular contexts. Tony responded favorably to the advice and expressed an interest in applying what he learned to the upcoming occasions.

TROUBLESHOOTING STICKY SITUATIONS

This section describes some of the more challenging clinical situations we have encountered in our work with college students, in addition to some recommended strategies.

Working with "Bravado" Drinkers

We have occasionally encountered students who boast repeatedly about their heavy drinking during the course of BASICS, recounting episodes of excessive drinking with pleasure. For these precontemplative and resistant individuals, significant negative consequences of drinking are described as if they were trophies or great feats. Although a therapist must be careful not to alienate such a student, it is important to gently display concern about the disparity between the risks and negative consequences described and the student's nonchalant affect. Depending on the degree of rapport established between the student and therapist, and on the therapist's clinical intuition, the approach to be taken in this type of situation will vary. We advise therapists to handle these situations cautiously and conservatively. It is far more important to avoid alienating the student (and, in so doing, to keep the door open for the student to seek services in the future) than to "prove a point." Stated somewhat differently, the broader goal of moving the client along the stages-of-change continuum—in this case, from precontemplation to contemplation—should always take precedence over all other specific goals or objectives.

Consider the following case: During the course of the brief intervention, Lisa described his parents and siblings as all having histories of alcohol problems. Although she mentioned the many ways in which their lives had been seriously compromised by their misuse of alcohol (e.g., marital difficulties between the parents, siblings' divorces, numerous legal and employment problems, several alcohol-related accidents, etc.), Lisa's tone of voice and affect in describing their circumstances had a proud, defiant quality. Lisa too had experienced numerous costly consequences of heavy drinking, including an arrest for drunk driving a few years back.

In this situation, the therapist had to decide the extent to which Lisa could be given feedback about the disparity between the risks and negative experiences she described and her proud affect. Two approaches were possible. Taking a more conservative tack, the therapist might have stated sometime during the interview, "We've been discussing some ways in which your drinking may be risky. How would you know if your use of alcohol became a problem? Specifically, what kinds of things would be likely to alert you to these problems?" The goal here would be to gently encourage Lisa in thinking about ways to recognize a problem. Should the student state an extreme consequence (e.g., "I would fail my courses because of alcohol") as the warning signal that alcohol problems might exist, the therapist could follow up with the following remark: "Hmm. It seems that by that time, the negative consequences would have become fairly extreme. I wonder what you might notice earlier that could serve as an alert signal."

In contrast to the approach described above, a more directive statement might be pursued:

> "You know, on other occasions when students have described similar family and personal situations as you have described just now to me, they generally express a great deal of concern. I noticed that when you described the kinds of problems your family members have had to face due to alcohol use, you didn't seem so concerned. I was curious about that." (*Pause for response*)

As previously mentioned, if in doubt a therapist should proceed with caution, remembering that the goal in all circumstances is to move the client forward along the stages-of-change continuum.

Working with Sanctioned Students

It is quite often the case that students are referred for special alcohol education workshops or counseling because of violations of campus policies involving alcohol. Although in theory this seems to be a practical and useful solution to a discipline problem, working with students who are mandated to participate poses special clinical challenges that must be addressed if the brief intervention is to have any impact on these students' behavior.

Typically, a student who is required to attend BASICS enters the first session resistant and angry. We believe that it is often best to address this issue in a gentle yet direct fashion. Unless these underlying feelings are addressed, it is likely that the student will either resist throughout the sessions or comply only to the extent that the requirement is fulfilled. Empathizing with the student's frustration can often result in the student's untangling the therapist from his or her anger at the administration or the arresting officer. In preparing the ground for working with a sanctioned student, it is usually important for the student to perceive the therapist as an ally and not as another disciplinarian.

In setting the stage for the sessions, the therapist should plan to address this issue at the outset; the degree of attention afforded to this topic depends largely on the response of the student and on the therapist's intuitive sense that reactance caused by mandating the session has dissipated. Early in the meeting and before assessment information is gathered, the therapist might ask the student to describe the circumstances that necessitated the interview. The therapist might then state, "So it sounds like this is something that you are being required to do rather than something you decided to do for yourself. Is that right?" Following a reply, the therapist might then ask the student to describe how he or she feels about this requirement. Depending on the student's responses, the therapist can always make use of identification as a tactic by stating,

> "You know, it is often difficult for us as therapists to be put in the position of providing these services to students who would normally otherwise decline. For our purposes here, I will not ask you to do anything that you do not want to do. Ultimately, what you do with the information will be entirely up to you."

By sharing his or her own feelings of frustration in this manner, the therapist is able to begin building a therapeutic alliance with the student as a means of working through this resistance.

Reactant Abstinence

We occasionally meet a student who has a considerable history of excessive drinking but who has endured or witnessed a significant consequence or tragedy due to alcohol and has thus decided to abstain from drinking completely. Such occasions have included experiencing a serious overdose requiring emergency room treatment, having a friend die of an alcohol overdose, and being sexually assaulted while intoxicated.

Consider the case of Mark, a college freshman living in a fraternity house. Prior to attending college, Mark had never tried alcohol. He stated that while he was in high school, he mostly associated with a studious group of students who "never partied." Shortly after moving into the fraternity, Mark began drinking on weekends with his peers. On one occasion (apparently his first occasion drinking hard alcohol), Mark consumed 30 shots in approximately 15 minutes. According to Mark, when he didn't feel buzzed after several minutes, he drank more. Mark recalled going to a basketball game with his fraternity brothers shortly after drinking. His next memory was of waking up in a hospital emergency room. He recalled, "My best friend was standing over me when I awoke, looking worried. He asked me why I had done what I did." Feeling scared and humiliated, Mark decided to move out of the fraternity house and move into the home of his uncle who lived near the university. He also decided to abstain from all alcohol use in the future.

Many therapists might have been inclined to congratulate Mark (an underage drinker) on his decision not to drink alcohol, without discussing further Mark's reasons for this decision or how he intended to carry it out. It would seem that Mark's decision was quite logical, given that his alcohol-related risk was eliminated so long as he continued to abstain. The weakest link in such a chain of logic is the potential for subsequent risk should an individual like Mark "relapse" or decide to abandon the goal of abstinence as the psychological trauma induced by the precipitating event wanes.

Our approach with these students is to support their goal of abstinence while recognizing that they may resume drinking in the near future if their fears about alcohol lessen. To support the goal of maintenance, we focus on developing skillful behaviors for use in situations where the students find it difficult to abstain or to have a good time while not drinking alcohol. We tell the students openly that these same skills can be used if they should begin to use alcohol again. If it seems likely from comments made by the students that they are likely to return to alcohol use in the near future, we may introduce moderation strategies while emphasizing again (particularly for underage drinkers) that the decision not to drink, at least for now, seems like a wise decision.

APPENDIX A

Discussion of Assessment Instruments Relevant to BASICS

*A*ppendix A discusses the instruments we have used in our research on college student's drinking to assess a variety of behavioral and psychological factors, including alcohol consumption and problems resulting from alcohol use, psychological distress, alcohol expectancies, life stress, eating habits, and use of other substances. Whereas many of the measures are well-established standardized measures, some of the measures were developed by our research team and are described here for the first time. Although this review is by no means exhaustive, the tools discussed here should provide a basis for therapists to construct their own assessment packages. Some of the measures described here are presented in Appendix D for readers' convenience.

ALCOHOL CONSUMPTION AND ALCOHOL-RELATED PROBLEMS[1]

Important guidelines to consider when assessing alcohol consumption include (1) using a standard measurement for drinks (e.g., 12 ounces of beer with 4% alcohol, 4 ounces of wine, 1¼ ounces of 80-proof spirits, etc.), and (2) determining the time frame involved in drinking (e.g., the number of hours over which the person consumed the drinks). When these two guidelines are used in combination, the assessor will have a more precise idea of a student's degree of intoxication. In addition, the assessment should obtain the following information about the student's **current** use of alcohol and related consequences:

- Information about current **typical pattern** (e.g., frequency of typical use, typical quantity of use).

---

[1] A thorough review of instruments used for assessing alcohol consumption and problems due to alcohol can be found in *Assessing Alcohol Problems* (NIAAA, 1995). In addition to including a number of measures in their entirety, this text includes excellent critiques of the various measures, as well as recommendations for their use. A copy of this document can be obtained from NIAAA through the National Clearinghouse for Alcohol and Drug Abuse.

• • •

- Information (e.g., frequency and quantity consumed) about recent **episodic occasions** over the last 30–90 days (30 days is the time period we generally assess, but a period of up to 90 days can be examined) when the student had more to drink than the typical pattern.

- **Negative outcomes** or events the student has experienced over the same period (see above) as a result of drinking.

Because problems due to drinking may be manifested in different ways by women and men, use of measures that include gender-specific as well as gender-neutral behaviors may be of importance (Dimeff et al., 1994). For example, men may be more likely to experience "public" or "external" consequences (e.g., getting into fights and damaging property) than women, and women may be more likely to experience "private" or "internal" behaviors (e.g., vomiting, skipping meals to "save" calories for drinking, shame, and guilt) than men.

When time allows, it is also useful to collect information about the student's **history of alcohol use,** including a history of problems resulting from alcohol. The purpose of gathering historical information, particularly about problems from drinking, is primarily to assess the lifetime severity of problems (i.e., just how far the student has been willing or able to go with drinking). Several quick questions to assess this history include the following:

- "Thinking back over the years since you have been drinking, what would you say was the worst experience that you had that resulted from alcohol?"

- "In addition, what were the last two occasions when you experienced negative consequences from alcohol?"

- "In comparison to other periods of your life, would you say you are drinking more with than you have in the past, less, or about the same?"

Brief Drinker Profile

The Brief Drinker Profile (BDP; Miller & Marlatt, 1984) is a sophisticated interview method for assessing alcohol consumption that yields far more information than comparable paper-and-pencil methods. Because it is a comprehensive measure, no other assessment of consumption may be required for clinical purposes. In addition to assessing the typical pattern of use, this measure includes an assessment of episodic occasions and an assessment of the time frame spent drinking. Typical and peak blood alcohol estimates can be readily obtained through the standard data gathered. For purposes of our brief intervention research, we utilized only the portions of the BDP assessing typical pattern and episodic occasions (see Chapter 4, Figures 4.1 and 4.2). Time required: 10–15 minutes (typical and episodic portions only).

Daily Drinking Questionnaire

On the Daily Drinking Questionnaire (DDQ; Collins et al., 1985), respondents fill in a series of seven boxes indicating their typical pattern of alcohol use on each day of the week in the past month. The DDQ has been modified to include a second set of boxes for typical number of hours spent drinking for each day in a usual week; this modified form of the DDQ is presented in Appendix D. Time required: 3 minutes.

Frequency–Quantity Questionnaire

A number of frequency–quantity methods exist for quickly and crudely assessing a person's habit of drinking alcohol (Straus & Bacon, 1953; Cahalan & Cisin, 1968; Cahalan, Cisin, & Crossley, 1969; Armor, Pollich, & Stambul, 1978). Our Frequency–Quantity Questionnaire adapted from Cahalan and Cisin (1968) assesses the maximum quantity consumed on a single occasion during the past month, typical quantity for a weekend evening, and frequency of drinking over the past month of time. Response options are extended to 19 drinks or more to accommodate the very heavy drinking habits of some students. The Frequency–Quantity Questionnaire is presented in Appendix D. Time required: 2 minutes.

Rutgers Alcohol Problems Inventory

The Rutgers Alcohol Problems Inventory (RAPI; White & Labouvie, 1989) consists of 23 items and asks the respondent to indicate the number of times a particular behavior has occurred while drinking or as a result of drinking in the past 3 years. We have modified the retrospective recall window from 3 years to much briefer periods (typically 1, 3, or 6 months), to allow us to detect changes in behavior as a result of our brief interventions. A factor analysis of the RAPI, using data gathered from our own research with high-risk college drinkers, resulted in five factors that accounted for 58.5% of the total variance (Dimeff et al., 1994). These factors include the following that occur as a direct result of drinking: (1) concern about drinking, (2) irresponsibility and neglect, (3) symptoms of alcohol dependence, (4) interpersonal conflict, and (5) family conflict. Clinical feedback from the RAPI can be provided in one of several fashions: in simple binary form (i.e., behaviors are discussed as either experienced or not experienced), with frequency weights (i.e., most frequently experienced consequences are discussed before less frequent items), or with greater emphasis on items suggestive of alcohol dependence. We focus first on all items suggestive of alcohol dependence, followed by those items with the highest frequency rating. Time required: 5 minutes.

Drinker Inventory of Consequences

The Drinker Inventory of Consequences (DrInC; Miller, Tonigan, & Longabaugh, 1995; Tonigan & Miller, 1993) is a self-administered 50-item questionnaire designed to assess negative consequences of alcohol abuse in five domains: intrapersonal physical, social, impulsive, and interpersonal. Like many other problem inventories, the DrInC is normed on adult samples. A particularly nice feature of this test is its use of lifetime experience, in addition to whether the behaviors were experienced in the past 3 months. Respondents are also asked how often they experienced a particular experience in the past 3 months. Time required: 10 minutes.

Young Adult Alcohol Problems Screening Test

The Young Adult Alcohol Problems Screening Test (YAAPST; Hurlbut & Sher, 1992) is a 27-item measure that assesses negative consequences from alcohol use over the student's lifetime and the past year, including the frequency of these behaviors. Like the RAPI, the YAAPST includes traditional consequences (e.g., hangovers, blackouts, driving while intoxicated), in addition to consequences unique to college students (e.g., missing classes, damaging property, involvement in regrettable sexual situations). Time required: 5–10 minutes.

Modified Sexual Experiences Survey

Based on Koss and colleagues' original survey for their national prevalence research on date rape (Koss & Oros, 1982), the modified Sexual Experiences Survey (Norris et al., 1996) is a 5-item measure that assesses sexual assault, including coercion, attempted rape and rape, and whether alcohol had been consumed prior to the assault. Time required: 5 minutes.

Brief Sexual Behaviors Survey

The Brief Sexual Behaviors Survey (BSBS) was developed for purposes of our research to assess sexual behaviors, including number and gender of sexual partners, condom use, and other (safe or risky) sex practices. The survey also includes questions about use of alcohol and other drugs during sexual intercourse. The BSBS is presented in Appendix D. Time required: 3 minutes.

ALCOHOL DEPENDENCE

Alcohol dependence can consist of three sets of processes: cognitive (e.g., believing that alcohol is required to get by, ruminating on the need for alcohol), behavioral (e.g., loss of control over drinking once initiation of drinking has begun), and/or physiological (e.g., tolerance, withdrawal, and "DTs"). For diagnostic purposes, alcohol dependence may best be assessed via a structured interview, such as the SCID (see below). Paper-and-pencil measures for assessing alcohol dependence can also produce highly reliable and valid results without additional interview time. Information about alcohol dependence can be useful as compelling motivational feedback underscoring the need for change; it is also essential for determining an appropriate drinking recommendation. For example, although we generally support moderation goals with our student clients, we do encourage abstinence for those with moderate to severe dependence on alcohol.

Alcohol Dependence Scale

The Alcohol Dependence Scale (ADS; Skinner & Horn, 1984) is a 25-item quantitative measure of alcohol dependence that covers cognitive, physiological, and behavioral domains, including withdrawal symptoms, impaired control while drinking, compulsion to drink, and prominence of drink-seeking behaviors. Several times ask the respondent about lifetime experiences related to alcohol dependence. This widely used measure is highly reliable and valid. The 12-month assessment window can be altered for a briefer time frame if used as an outcome measure. Time required: 5 minutes.

Structured Clinical Interview for DSM-IV Axis I Disorders

The Patient Edition of the Structured Clinical Interview for DSM-IV Axis I Disorders (SCID; First et al., 1995) includes a total of 22 structured questions that cover the DSM-IV diagnostic criteria for substance abuse and substance dependence. A frequently used instrument in clinical research, the SCID has sound psychometric properties. Time required: 5–15 minutes.

FAMILY HISTORY OF ALCOHOL OR OTHER SUBSTANCE USE PROBLEMS

Donovan (1995) has noted that family history of alcohol or other substance use problems may function as an individual risk factor in one of several ways (e.g., Schuckit, 1991; Tarter, 1991). Young adults with a positive family history may have stronger alcohol expectancies that interact with the individuals' drinking behavior (e.g., Brown, Craemer, & Stetson, 1987; Mann, Cassin, & Sher, 1987; Sher et al., 1991). Persons with a positive family history may also have a fundamentally different developmental course of problems, different pattern of drinking, and poorer treatment prognosis than individuals without a positive family history (Babor, Bolinsky, et al., 1992; Litt, Babor, DelBoca, Kadden, & Cooney, 1992). We review family history of alcohol and other substance use problems within the brief intervention under the rubric of "individual risk factors" that may predispose the student to alcohol or drug problems.

There is no gold standard for how to quantify or interpret an individual's degree of risk for alcohol problems on the basis of family history. For sake of ease in providing graphic feedback, we have elected to use the quantitative method of counting up the total number of relatives identified as a having a drinking problem (regardless of severity). We created three classes of risk due to genetic predisposition to alcohol problems: "strongly positive," to designate risk for students with two or more relatives with problem drinking histories; "positive," for students having one relative with a history of drinking problems; and "negative," for students identifying no family members with problem drinking histories.

Adapted Short Michigan Alcoholism Screening Test

The Adapted Short Michigan Alcoholism Screening Test (Sher & Descutner, 1986) is a self-administered test that is an adaptation of the Short Michigan Alcoholism Screening Test (SMAST; Selzer, Vinokur, & van Rooijen, 1976). There are two separate measures, one for fathers (Adapted SMAST for fathers; F-SMAST) and another for mothers (Adapted SMAST for mothers; M-SMAST), each containing 13 yes–no items about the parent's drinking behavior and experience of negative consequences from alcohol. Time required: 5 minutes.

Addiction Severity Index

The Addiction Severity Index (ASI; McLellan, Luborsky, O'Brien, & Woody, 1980; McLellan et al., 1992) is a structured interview that includes a brief family history of alcohol and other drug problems. The interviewer asks, "Have any of your relatives had what you would call a significant drinking, drug use, or psychological problem—one that did or should have led to treatment?" Miller et al. (1992) utilized this section of the ASI in providing feedback to patients in the motivational interviewing treatment condition in their research. Points were assigned for each relative, using the following codes when a relative was positive for alcohol or drug problems: add 2 points for each positive mother, father, sister, and/or brother; add 1 point for each positive grandparent or uncle/aunt. Family risk classification codes were as follows: low risk (0–1); medium risk (2–3), high risk (4–6), and very high risk (7+).

Family Tree Questionnaire

The Family Tree Questionnaire (Mann et al., 1985) is an easy-to-use assessment measure that provides respondents with a family tree diagram, which furnishes a consistent set of cues for identifying blood relatives with alcohol problems. This measure can be either administered during an interview or self-administered. Respondents are asked to classify each relative in one of the following categories: (1) "never drank," (2) "social drinker," (3) "possible problem drinker," (4) "definite problem drinker," (5) "no relatives" (for cases where a respondent is an only child), or (6) "don't know/don't remember." Time required: About 5–10 minutes.

MEDICAL SCREENING

The primary medical assessment that is indicated for young adult drinkers is a screening for the presence of medical conditions in which use of alcohol is contraindicated. The most common medical conditions presented by heavy-drinking students are ulcers, liver damage or dysfunction, or diabetes. On occasion, students are taking medications that are potentiated or compromised by the use of alcohol. Because of alcohol's known effects on pregnancy and the fetus (see Streissguth, 1983; Streissguth, Barr, Sampson, & Bookstein, 1994), we always inquire about whether a woman is pregnant or has any reason to suspect she may be pregnant. Complete abstinence from all use of alcohol is always recommended for pregnant or possibly pregnant women. We routinely ask the following questions:

- "Has a physician ever recommended that you cut down or not drink alcohol?"

- "Are you currently being treated for any medical conditions, or are you taking any medications?"

- For women: "Are you pregnant, or do you have any reason to believe you might be pregnant?"

ALCOHOL EXPECTANCIES

The term **alcohol expectancies** typically refers to beliefs an individual holds about the anticipated effects or outcomes of consuming alcohol, which are usually shaped through the process of direct and indirect experiences with alcohol and drinking behavior (Donovan, 1995). Most simply, alcohol expectancies may be thought of as the reasons why people drink. In a clinical context, therapists can work to decrease positive alcohol expectancies as a means of decreasing actual drinking behavior. Within the context of BASICS, we first discuss the concept of alcohol expectancies by reviewing the positive alcohol expectancies endorsed by the student, followed by an attempt at challenging the factual validity of the expectancy with data from the balanced-placebo research on the actual effects of alcohol. An alcohol expectancy measure can also be used as an outcome measure, to determine whether the student's cognitive expectancies have shifted in a favorable (less positive) direction as a result of the intervention.

Comprehensive Effects of Alcohol

The Comprehensive Effects of Alcohol (CEA) survey (Fromme et al., 1993) is a 38-item self-administered questionnaire that assesses positive as well as negative drinking expectancies. Positive expectancy factors include sociability, tension reduction, "liquid courage," and sexuality. Negative factors include cognitive and behavioral impairment, risk and aggression, and self-perception. Items focus on specific discrete effects of alcohol. Respondents first indicate on a 4-point scale whether they agree or disagree with a particular belief. A rating of the perceived effect's desirability is then assigned on a 5-point scale. Positive alcohol outcome expectancies are those rated likely to occur and perceived as desirable. When summarizing the results of the CEA as part of the graphic feedback material in our research, we selected the five most salient positive expectancies. The CEA is presented in Appendix D. Time required: 5–10 minutes.

MOTIVATION TO CHANGE

Measures assessing a student's motivation to change can be used as outcome measures, as well as clinical tools that permit the therapist to determine anticipate the student's interest in making changes in his or her use of alcohol.

Readiness to Change Questionnaire

The Readiness to Change Questionnaire (RTCQ; Rollnick, Heather, Gold, & Hall, 1992) is a self-administered 12-item questionnaire based on Prochaska and DiClemente's stages-of-change model. Three subscales that correspond to three stages in this model (Precontemplation, Contemplation, Action) are generated by the RTCQ, which ultimately determines the respondent's stage of change. Respondents provide responses to each item on a 5-point Likert scale. Time required: About 3 minutes.

University of Rhode Island Change Assessment

The University of Rhode Island Change Assessment (URICA; McConnaughy, Prochaska, & Velicer, 1983) includes 32 items, each of which is responded to on a 5-point Likert scale (from "strong disagreement" to "strong agreement"). Results indicate a respondent's stage of change, again according to Prochaska and DiClemente's stages-of-change model. Four stages of change are assessed by the URICA: precontemplation, contemplation, action, and maintenance. Time required: About 8 minutes.

LIFE STRESS AND PSYCHOLOGICAL DISTRESS

Although heavy drinking is generally not associated with psychological distress in college students (as it often is for older adults), a small percentage of students nonetheless do use alcohol as a means of reducing anxiety and depression or of coping with inordinate life stress. In some of these cases, students report having frequent thoughts about killing themselves— perhaps as the ultimate escape from pressures and despair. For these reasons, we typically include a self-administered assessment of life stress and psychological distress when time allows. To the extent that these problems are linked to or exacerbated by alcohol use, we discuss these links during the feedback session.

Brief Symptom Inventory

The Brief Symptom Inventory (BSI; Derogatis & Spencer, 1982), an abridged version of the Symptom Checklist 90 (Derogatis, 1977), is a 49-item behavioral instrument that assesses eight psychological distress dimensions and provides several indices by which to measure general symptoms of distress. The eight clinical dimensions are as follows: depression, anxiety, hostility, obsessive–compulsive symptoms, paranoid ideation, somatization, phobic anxiety, and psychoticism. Global indices of functioning include the Global Severity Index (which combines information on the number of symptoms endorsed and the intensity of the endorsement to yield the most single most sensitive indicator of distress), the Positive Symptom Distress Index (which measures pure intensity, "corrected" for the number of symptoms positively endorsed), and the Positive Symptoms Total (which provides the number of symptoms reported by the patient). Time required: 5–10 minutes.

Life Experiences Survey

The Life Experiences Survey (LES; Sarason et al., 1978) consists of a list of 60 common stress-producing events. Respondents are asked to indicate those they have experienced in the last year and to rate the degree of stress they experienced as a result of each event. In addition to its established use for research and clinical purposes, the LES is fairly comprehensive in its inclusion of stressful life events. Because the LES was developed for use primarily with older adults, some of the questions are not relevant for younger audiences. Time required: 10–15 minutes.

RISK PERCEPTION

We have found it useful to know something about how the student views his or her risks before entering into the feedback and advice session of BASICS, particularly when there is a large disparity between the student's perceived risk and report of actual recent problems from drinking too much (this usually takes the form of a low risk perception and a high report of problems). Having information about a disparity between actual and perceived risk can be useful in considering approaches for the session, to ensure that defensiveness is minimized. In these cases, there may be more of a need to emphasize basic information about alcohol and the possible risks of heavy alcohol use. We have found that providing these students with feedback about the disparity between their perception and experience can serve as a "wake-up call." For those who are inclined to evaluate their risks from drinking more accurately, this feedback can be experienced as validating.

Alcohol Perceived Risks Assessment

The 16-item self-administered Alcohol Perceived Risks Assessment (APRA; Duthie et al., 1991) assesses the degree of college students' perceived likelihood of experiencing problems from heavy drinking over the course of their years at college. Students use a 7-point scale to rate how likely they are to experience a particular negative consequence (e.g., hangovers, getting into fights, etc.) due to drinking. A comparison can then be made between a student's perception of risk as reported by the APRA and data from other measures (e.g., the RAPI) on actual negative consequences the student has reported experiencing, as described above. Data from the APRA can also be considered against the student's motivation to change (e.g., low perception of risk and low motivation to change, accurate perception of risk based on current experience of negative consequences and high motivation to change, etc.). The APRA is presented in Appendix D. Time required: 4 minutes.

PERCEPTIONS OF NORMATIVE DRINKING BEHAVIOR

Research on perceived norms has documented that heavy-drinking students view their drinking habits as fairly representative of general college norms (Baer & Carney, 1993; Baer et al., 1991). This is not all that surprising, given that people typically associate with others who are like themselves, with similar interests and habits. As a result, students may develop a false sense that their drinking habits are well within the average range, when in fact they may dramatically exceed the norm. This belief can serve as a risk factor for problems associated with alcohol. Gathering this information can also serve as a "reality check" during the brief intervention.

Drinking Norms Rating Form

Developed by Baer et al. (1991), the Drinking Norms Rating Form (DNRF) specifically asks the student to indicate how much and how often a typical college student drinks, and how much and how often students residing in different settings (e.g., a fraternity or sorority, a residence hall, an off-campus residence, with parents, etc.) drink. If the student's perception of college drinking norms is significantly inaccurate, it can be challenged during the feedback session on the basis of normative data. The DNRF is presented in Appendix D. Time required: 5 minutes.

EATING HABITS

The incidence of disordered eating among college women is alarmingly high, and eating disturbances often overlap with heavy alcohol use (Krahn, 1991; Yeary & Heck, 1989).

Eating Attitudes Test—26

The Eating Attitudes Test—26 (EAT-26; Garner, Olmsted, Bohr, & Garfinkel, 1982) is a widely used 26-item self-administered questionnaire normed on inpatient women with eating disorders. Six response points per item range from "never" to "always." The EAT-26 has three subscales: Dieting, Bulimia and Food Preoccupation, and Oral Control. For scoring purposes, low-base-rate responses (including "rarely" and "sometimes," along with "never") are scored as 0. Only high-base-rate behaviors (e.g., "often," "very often," or "always") receive scores greater than 0 (specifically, 1, 2, and 3, respectively). Low base rates are utilized to assess for less severely problematic eating. Time required: 5–10 minutes.

Disordered Eating Questionnaire

We developed the Disordered Eating Questionnaire to assess the frequency of a student's dieting, binge eating, use of diet pills, use of laxatives, and self-induced vomiting over the past 3 months. This measure also includes segments of an instrument developed by Meilman et al. (1991) to assess the number of occasions in the past 3 months a student has self-induced vomiting after drinking alcohol and eating. Time required: 5 minutes.

PRIOR HISTORY OF BEHAVIORAL PROBLEMS

One of the best predictors of alcohol problems in young adults—perhaps second only to current drinking habits and problems resulting from drinking—is a prior history of behavioral problems, especially when such a history qualifies for a formal DSM-IV diagnosis of conduct disorder. Students who have a history of numerous behavioral problems during childhood and adolescence are more likely to have continued behavioral problems across a number of behavioral domains (including alcohol and other substance use problems) in young adulthood (Jessor & Jessor, 1977; Jessor, 1991, 1993). Although this trend is particularly robust among males, rates of alcohol abuse are also higher among females with a history of conduct disorder than among females without this history (Heath, Bucholz, Madden, et al., 1997). In our recent Lifestyles Project, drinkers who met DSM-III-R criteria for conduct disorder (according to their self-report of behavioral problems before the age of 17) were more likely to report recent alcohol problems than drinkers who did not meet these criteria. Put simply, behavioral problems predict other behavioral problems. Data from an assessment of prior history of behavioral problems can be used to identify students who may be at greater risk for alcohol problems. This information can also be used for motivational feedback to alert students of their risk.

Structured Clinical Interview for DSM-IV Axis I Disorders

The Patient Edition of the SCID (First et al., 1995), previously discussed in regard to alcohol dependence, also includes a series of structured questions that cover the DSM-IV diagnostic criteria for conduct disorder.

APPENDIX B

Personalized Graphic Feedback and "Tips" Sheets

PERSONALIZED GRAPHIC FEEDBACK

As we have described in Chapter 5 of this manual, we provide each of our student participants with a personalized graphic feedback sheet during the second session of BASICS. The key to success with such a graphic is the "personalization"—that is, the customizing of message and content to the needs, the habits, and (to the extent possible) the style of the participant for whom the material is intended. In this part of Appendix B, we present an example of a feedback sheet we developed for BASICS, as well as an example of a "booster" feedback sheet developed for a later stage of our longitudinal research.

BASICS Personalized Graphic Feedback

Figures B.1, B.2, and B.3 (B.1 and B.2 are closeups that highlight the components; B.3 shows the sheet as a whole) depict the personalized graphic feedback sheet we designed for the form of BASICS we tested in our Lifestyles Project. This sheet emphasizes the student's drinking habits relative to those of other students, as well as the student's individual risk factors. Although this particular graphic does not contain individualized messages that comment on the data, such messages might further enhance its appeal and effectiveness. The layout of this graphic allowed it to serve as a visual outline for discussion during the second session of BASICS.

"Booster" Personalized Graphic Feedback

Each student in our Lifestyles Project completed a yearly assessment packet, which was mailed to the student's home and was later used to generate subsequent personalized graphics. These "booster" graphics (see Figure B.4 for an example) typically depicted changes in the student's use of alcohol and related problems, using various bar charts and histograms. In addition to this visual representation of changes over time, we included several personalized motivational

• • •

Personal Feedback for John Student Drinker
Student's Name

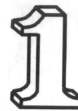

Your Drinking Patterns

- *Frequency*
- *Quantity*
- *Percentile Comparison*
- *Blood Alcohol Content*

FALL TERM 1990
Frequency/
Quantity during
Fall

According to the information you gave us during the Fall 1990 Assessment, the **number of occasions you drank (frequency) was 3 - 4 times a week**. The **average amount you drank on each occasion (quantity) was 5 - 6 drinks**. Your percentile rank (comparing you to other college students) is **91%**.

Percentile Rating

Your **typical peak blood alcohol content (BAC)** in the Fall term was **.117**. Your **highest reported BAC** in the Fall Assessment was **.238**.

Peak BAL during
Fall
Highest Peak BAL

SPRING SEMESTER IN HIGH SCHOOL
Frequency/
Quantity during
High School

During the final semester in high school, your **frequency** of drinking was 1 - 2 times a week, and the average **quantity** you consumed on each occasion was 3 - 4 drinks.

DRINKING NORMS
Perceived Norms

In the fall, you filled out questions about **what you believed to be the average frequency and quantity of alcohol consumed by other students** your age. You told us that you believed that the average student drank 1 - 2 times each week and during each occasion, s/he consumed 5 - 6 drinks.

The **actual drinking norm** for adults your age is **twice a week**, drinking about **four drinks on each occasion**.

Actual Norms

	FREQUENCY	QUANTITY	PEAK BAC	
Current				
Fall 1990	**3 - 4/wk.**	**5 - 6 drinks**	**N/A**	Summary
Spring 1990	1 - 2/wk.	3 - 4 drinks	N/A	
Actual Student Norm	2/wk.	4 drinks	N/A	
Your Estimated Norm	1 - 2/wk.	5 - 6 drinks	N/A	

FIGURE B.1. Personalized graphic feedback sheet for the form of BASICS tested in the Life-styles project, 1990–1991: Closeup of left side, with components highlighted.

· · ·

Lifestyles

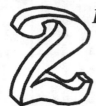 *Risks*

- *Alcohol-Related Consequences*
- *Family History*
- *Dependence*
- *Beliefs*

ALCOHOL-RELATED CONSEQUENCES

Alcohol-related
Problems (RAPI)

From the information we gathered during the Fall Assessments, you indicated that the following alcohol-related consequences had occurred at least three to five times in the prior six months:

- Not able to do your homework or study for a test.
- Got into fights, acted bad, or did mean things.
- Caused shame or embarrassment to someone.
- Felt that you needed more alcohol than you used to use in order to get the same effect.
- Noticed a change in your personality.
- Missed a day (or part of a day) of school or work.

FAMILY HISTORY

Family History

From the information you gave us, we consider your risk based on family history to be **strongly positive.**

INDICES OF ALCOHOL DEPENDENCE

Alcohol
Dependency

In your personal interview you acknowledged the following experiences which are associated with a pattern of dependence:

- Being intoxicated or hungover when at work, school, or driving.
- Giving up other activities to drink.
- Drinking more than you intended.

BELIEFS ABOUT ALCOHOL AND ITS EFFECTS

Beliefs about
Alcohol

You listed the following alcohol effects as "Good" and "Likely to Occur" when you consume alcohol:

- I would be outgoing.
- I would be brave and daring.
- I would feel calm.
- I would be a better lover.
- It would be easier to act out my fantasies.

- I would be humorous.
- I would feel sexy.
- I would take risks.
- I would feel calm.

Your concern about your drinking habits is **moderate** and your perceived risk for alcohol-related consequences is **considerable.**

Concern about
Drinking Habits

Perceived Risk

FIGURE B.2. Personalized graphic feedback sheet for the form of BASICS tested in the Lifestyles project, 1990–1991: Closeup of right side, with components highlighted.

Lifestyles

Personal Feedback for John Student Drinker

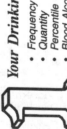

Your Drinking Patterns

- Frequency
- Quantity
- Percentile Comparison
- Blood Alcohol Content

FALL TERM 1990

According to the information you gave us during the Fall 1990 Assessment, the **number of occasions you drank (frequency) was 3 - 4 times a week.** The **average amount you drank on each occasion (quantity) was 5 - 6 drinks.** Your percentile rank (comparing you to other college students) is **91%.**

Your **typical peak blood alcohol content (BAC)** in the Fall term was **.117.** Your **highest reported BAC** in the Fall Assessment was **.238.**

SPRING SEMESTER IN HIGH SCHOOL

During the final semester in high school, your **frequency** of drinking was 1 - 2 times a week, and the average **quantity** you consumed on each occasion was 3 - 4 drinks.

DRINKING NORMS

In the fall, you filled out questions about **what you believed to be the average frequency and quantity of alcohol consumed by other students** your age. You told us that you believed that the average student drank 1 - 2 times each week and during each occasion, s/he consumed 5 - 6 drinks.

The **actual drinking norm** for adults your age is **twice a week,** drinking about **four drinks on each occasion.**

Current	FREQUENCY	QUANTITY	PEAK BAC
Fall 1990	3 - 4/wk.	5 - 6 drinks	N/A
Spring 1990	1 - 2/wk.	3 - 4 drinks	N/A
Actual Student Norm	2/wk.	4 drinks	N/A
Your Estimated Norm	1 - 2/wk.	5 - 6 drinks	N/A

Risks

- Alcohol-Related Consequences
- Family History
- Dependence
- Beliefs

ALCOHOL-RELATED CONSEQUENCES

From the information we gathered during the Fall Assessments, you indicated that the following alcohol-related consequences had occurred at least three to five times in the prior six months:

- Not able to do your homework or study for a test.
- Got into fights, acted bad, or did mean things.
- Caused shame or embarrassment to someone.
- Felt that you needed more alcohol than you used to use in order to get the same effect.
- Noticed a change in your personality.
- Missed a day (or part of a day) of school or work.

FAMILY HISTORY

From the information you gave us, we consider your risk based on family history to be **strongly positive.**

INDICES OF ALCOHOL DEPENDENCE

In your personal interview you acknowledged the following experiences which are associated with a pattern of dependence:

- Being intoxicated or hungover when at work, school, or driving.
- Giving up other activities to drink.
- Drinking more than you intended.

BELIEFS ABOUT ALCOHOL AND ITS EFFECTS

You listed the following alcohol effects as "Good" and "Likely to Occur" when you consume alcohol:

- I would be outgoing.
- I would be brave and daring.
- I would feel calm.
- I would be a better lover.
- It would be easier to act out my fantasies.
- I would be humorous.
- I would feel sexy.
- I would take risks.
- I would feel calm.

Your concern about your drinking habits is **moderate** and your perceived risk for alcohol-related consequences is **considerable.**

FIGURE B.3. Personalized graphic feedback sheet for the form of BASICS tested in the Lifestyles project, 1990–1991.

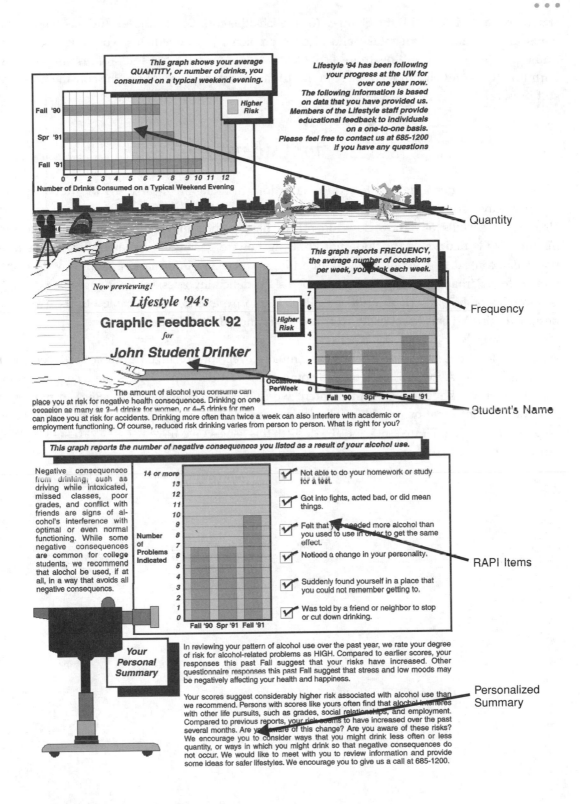

FIGURE B.4. "Booster" personalized graphic feedback sheet for a later stage of the Lifestyles project, fall, 1992, with components highlighted.

statements associated with the changes (or the lack thereof). For example, students who made gains in reducing alcohol intake and alcohol problems but nonetheless continued to report numerous problems resulting from alcohol use were congratulated for progress in reducing harmful effects and encouraged to continue striving for change, in light of the considerable risk still present.

"TIPS" SHEETS

Although motivational deficits to reduce hazardous drinking are clearly significant barriers to moving heavy drinkers into less risky drinking habits, we hypothesize that many young adults also lack the skills or "know-how" to make changes they may otherwise be interested in making. Skills deficits can include not knowing how to generate a behavioral response in a particular context (e.g., drink refusal), in addition to lacking information about how to drink more safely. Perhaps the clearest example of a skills deficit involves not knowing when enough is enough—or how much alcohol it really takes to experience pleasurable effects. We have designed "tips" sheets specifically to address this and other skills deficits.

We generate a separate "tips" sheet to accompany every personalized graphic feedback sheet students receive. Although the look and some of the content "tips" sheets have changed from year to year, we have repeated the content we find essential: specific strategies to moderate alcohol use, information about alcohol expectancies, and information about the biphasic response to alcohol. Figures B.5 and B.6 depict "tips" sheets we have used at various stages of our research.

Tips for Reduced Lifestyle Risk from Alcohol

You can have a good time
without drinking,
or, if you choose,
while consuming
alcohol
in a lower-risk manner.

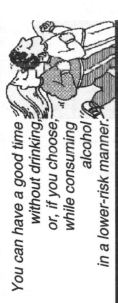

Consider what you WANT

For those who are not *tolerant*, alcohol effects are a function of blood alcohol level:

.02% Non-tolerant drinkers begin to feel some effect (about one drink).

.04% Most people begin to feel relaxed.

.06% Judgment is somewhat impaired; people are less able to make rational decisions about their capabilities, for example, driving.

.08% Definite impairment of muscle coordination and driving skills. Increased risk of nausea and slurred speech.

.10% Clear deterioration of reaction time and control. *Legal intoxication.*

.15% Balance and movement are impaired. Risk of blackouts and accidents.

.30% Many people lose consciousness. Risk of death.

Consider HOW you drink

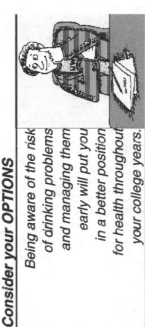

Biphasic Response to Alcohol

Euphoria-up

FEELING
SCALE 0

Downhome-
down

tolerance
develops

TIME

After

More alcohol may **not** give you more of what you want. Most adults drink for a mild effect but avoid painful and dangerous side effects. The more and faster you drink, the *less* you will experience mild stimulating effects and the *more* you will feel depressant effects.

Tolerance is a risk factor for alcohol problems (academic, legal social, and health). It overrides nature's way of telling you that you have had too much. It makes drinking more expensive and decreases enjoyment of mild effects.

Consider MYTHS and REALITY

Alcohol's effects on social behavior often come more from culture than from chemistry. In fact, the belief that one has consumed alcohol is sufficient for most people to feel more relaxed, at ease, confident, or sexual. This is true even if the person has not actually had any alcohol, but simply thinks that they have. The chemical effects of alcohol slow motor coordination and skill, and can impact thinking and judgment.

Consider your OPTIONS

Being aware of the risk
of drinking problems
and managing them
early will put you
in a better position
for health throughout
your college years.

Specific Tips for Reduced Risk Drinking

*   Have fun without drinking.
*   If you choose to drink, drink slowly.
*   Keep track of how much you drink.
*   Eat before drinking.
*   Space your drinks.
*   Alternate alcoholic drinks with non-alcoholic beverages.
*   Drink for quality rather than quantity.
*   Set a limit based on BAL not over .05%.
*   Avoid drinking games.
*   Be prepared to handle situations, people, and places where heavy drinking occurs.
*   Experiment with drinking less and refusing drinks.
*   Drink reduced alcohol beer instead of stronger spirits.

FIGURE B.5. "Tips" sheet, 1990–1991.

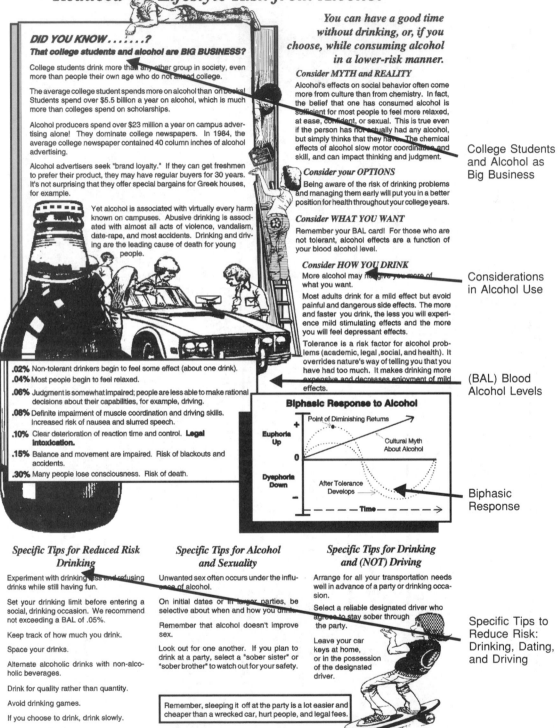

FIGURE B.6. "Tips" sheet, 1992, with components highlighted.

APPENDIX C

Harm Reduction Handouts for Students Who Drink

*I*n this appendix, we provide several handouts that can be reproduced from this manual and given to students who drink alcohol. These handouts were developed for distribution by medical care providers, in a separate research project involving high-risk drinkers who were receiving services at a student health primary care center (Dimeff, 1996). Many of the handouts include a motivational "grabber" ("Questions to Think About") and a simplified description of research findings ("Here's What We Learned" or "Here's What You Should Consider"). Handouts such as these can be used to further tailor or augment information from the "tips" sheet. The BASICS provider can personalize them by circling, highlighting, underlining, or otherwise marking directly on a particular student's copy to emphasize particularly relevant content for that student.

THINKING ABOUT MODERATING YOUR DRINKING?

Decide what you want from drinking alcohol.

- Think about the pros and cons (short- and long-term) for moderating your use versus maintaining the status quo.

- Also consider what you absolutely want to avoid when you drink.

Set drinking limits.

- What's your upper limit on the number of drinks you consume per week?

- At what point do you decide you've had enough (consider a BAL limit)?

- What's the maximum number of days for drinking you will choose to give yourself?

- Use standard guidelines to determine what constitutes one drink:

1¼ ounces of 80-proof spirits; 4 ounces of wine; 10 ounces of beer with 5% alcohol ("ice" beer and many "microbrews"); 12 ounces of beer with 4% alcohol (standard beer).

Count your drinks and monitor your drinking behavior.

- Try it! Most people are surprised by what they learn when they actually count how much they drink.

- Simply observe your behavior—this is like standing outside yourself and watching how you are acting when you are drinking.

Alter how and what you drink.

- Switch to drinks that contain less alcohol (e.g., light beers).

- Slow down your pace of drinking.

- Space drinks further apart.

- Alternate drinking nonalcoholic beverages with alcoholic drinks.

Manage your drinking in the moment.

- Stay awake and on top of how you drink and what you're drinking when you're at a party.

- Choose what's right for you.

POSITIVE ALCOHOL EXPECTANCIES

Questions to Think About:

- To what extent is people's experience after drinking alcohol psychological versus chemical?

- Is it possible to feel "buzzed," light-headed, and "tipsy" without drinking any alcohol?

What Are Positive Alcohol Expectancies?

- **Positive alcohol expectancies** are beliefs people have about what they will experience after drinking alcohol (e.g., "I'll feel more social and outgoing," "I'll feel more sexy and friendly").

What's the Balanced-Placebo Design and Why Is It So Important?

- The balanced-placebo design is a research design developed by Dr. G. Alan Marlatt at the University of Washington to test the extent to which people's experience after drinking alcohol is psychological versus pharmacological. In Marlatt's research, people were brought into his BARLAB, which looked like a real tavern.

- The research experimentally manipulated what a person believed he or she was drinking (expected alcohol or expected tonic water) and what he or she actually received (alcohol or tonic).

Balanced-Placebo Research Design

	Expected Alcohol	**Expected Tonic**
Received Alcohol	Person received what he or she expected (alcohol).	*"Spiked Drink"* Person received alcoholic beverage when he or she was expecting tonic water.
Received Tonic	*Placebo* Person received tonic water when he or she was expecting alcohol.	Person received what he or she expected (tonic water).

(p.1 of 2; continued)

• • •

Here's What We Learned:

1. Alcohol expectancies contributed powerfully to the "buzz" people often experienced after drinking, particularly when they drank lightly to moderately. The effect diminished with heavy drinking (over approximately 0.07% BAL).

2. A "buzz" was found to have **two ingredients**: (1) what people expected to happen, or their **mental set**; and (2) the environmental **setting** (e.g., dim lights, music, others drinking, a drink, having fun).

3. The **belief** alone that people had consumed alcohol could make them feel less socially inhibited.

4. Men often became less socially anxious when they believed they had consumed alcohol; women reported more social anxiety in the same condition.

5. Men typically experienced more sexual arousal when they believed they had consumed alcohol, even though actual physiological sexual response was dampened.

THE BIPHASIC RESPONSE
(OR "MORE ISN'T NECESSARILY BETTER")

Questions to Think About:

- Does "more" mean "better" when it comes to drinking alcohol?

- Why do you feel initially energized, but tired and wanting to crash later on, after you've been drinking for a while?

- What role does tolerance play in getting "high" from alcohol?

What Is the Biphasic Response?

- The **biphasic response** refers to the two physiological phases, or sets of effects, that alcohol produces. Feeling stimulated or excited is characteristic of the initial phase, followed by depressant effects, such as feeling tired.

- The initial positive effects are associated with low but rising BALs. The second-phase effects are associated more with falling BALs (regardless of your peak BAL, although the effects are more profound when the peak is higher).

Why Is the Biphasic Response Important?

- It allows you to test whether the conventional wisdom that "more" means "better" is really true or not.

- It helps you understand how tolerance affects you physiologically when it comes to drinking alcohol.

Here's What to Consider:

- As it turns out, if you want to hold onto a good buzz and not lose steam midway through a party, you're a lot better off drinking slowly and moderately (not pushing a BAL over **0.055%**) and getting rid of your tolerance.

- You're guaranteed a nasty hangover (one of the more unpleasant depressant effects) when you binge-drink (e.g., have a lot of drinks in a row, the way you may do if you play drinking games).

- The more alcohol you drink and the higher your BAL, the more alcohol acts as a depressant instead of as a stimulant.

- The **more** tolerance to alcohol you've got, the **less** likely you are to experience the stimulating physiological effects of alcohol.

ALCOHOL INTOXICATION AND PERFORMANCE

Questions to Think About:

- What effect does getting drunk on Wednesday have on your performance during Friday's game?

- You've got your midterm on Monday. Does it matter how much you drink on Saturday night?

Here Are the Simple Facts about Alcohol and Performance:

- Alcohol intoxication messes with your sleep!

- This limits your ability to think and respond quickly.

- In turn, your slower thinking and responding cut down on your ability to perform well.

Here Are the Technical Facts about Alcohol Intoxication and Sleep:

1. Alcohol intoxication increases total sleep time during the first half of the night, but decreases it during the second half of the night.

2. When you're intoxicated, you may sleep more soundly during the first half of the night; during the second half of the night, however, you'll sleep lightly and be easily woken.

3. Rapid eye movement (REM) decreases during the first half of the night after light to moderate drinking; this is followed by REM rebound during the second half of the night. **Heavy drinking, however, will compromise your REM throughout the night.**

4. It decreases the deep, restful part of the sleep cycle.

5. Physiologically, sleep deprivation results in the suppression of normal hormonal levels, which ultimately decreases your oxygen availability and consumption. All of this substantially decreases endurance, due to temporary impairment of the aerobic pathways.

Here's What You Should Consider:

- If you want a peak performance—whether it's in the classroom or on the playing field—either plan to abstain from alcohol use altogether before a big performance, or drink in moderation if you choose to drink.

- You can moderate your use of alcohol by not drinking past the point when you just begin to feel a mild buzz from the alcohol. This would be about **three drinks in 3 hours or four drinks in 5 hours for a 130-pound woman**, or **five drinks in 3 hours or six drinks in 5 hours for a 180-pound man.**

- Get good sleep.

GENDER DIFFERENCES AND ALCOHOL
(OR THE BIG GAP IN LEVELS OF INTOXICATION)

Questions to Think About:

- All things being equal, are women more likely to become intoxicated than men?

- Why do women get more intoxicated on alcohol at certain times of the month?

Here Are the Facts about Gender Differences and Alcohol:

- If a woman matches drinks with a male counterpart, she is likely to become significantly more intoxicated. This is true even when they weigh the same amount (see below).

- Some studies have found that people unwittingly tend to match drinking styles (e.g., amount, pace, etc.) when drinking together. Generally, men tend to be the pace setters when they are drinking with women.

- If you consider the usual weight differences for college women and men, a woman who drinks the same amount as a man will be nearly twice as intoxicated.

Here's Why:

1. **Men usually weigh a lot more than women.** The typical college man weighs 180 pounds, but the average college woman weighs approximately 130 pounds.

2. On average, a man's total body weight is composed of more water than a woman's (55–65% vs. 45–55%). The more water **in a person's body, the more alcohol gets diluted.**

3. Levels of **alcohol dehydrogenase,** a stomach enzyme that aids in the metabolism of alcohol before it enters the bloodstream (this is known as **first-pass metabolism**), are 70–80% higher in men than in women. These differences may make women more vulnerable to developing liver cirrhosis and cognitive impairment over time than men.

4. **Hormonal changes in women also affect BALs.** Studies have shown that women are likely to stay intoxicated for longer periods of time 1 week before and 1 week after menstruating.

5. Women who are using **oral contraceptives** are also likely to maintain the peak degree of intoxication for longer than they would otherwise. This prolonged peak appears related to an increase in estrogen levels.

(p. 1 of 2; continued)

• • •

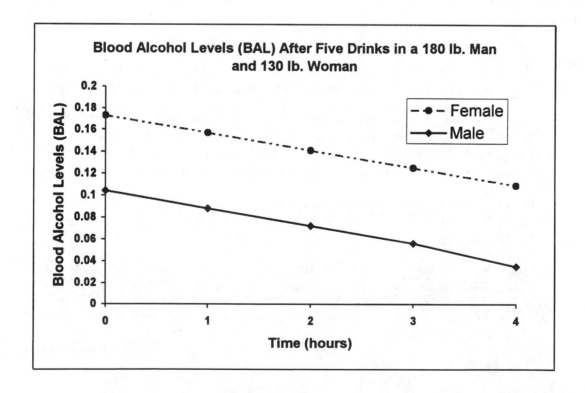

ALCOHOL AND SEXUAL ASSAULT

Questions to Think About:

- Does alcohol really increase a woman's risk of being sexually assaulted or raped?

- If alcohol really does increase the odds, how?

Here Are the Facts about Alcohol and Unwanted Sex:

In 1987, Dr. Mary Koss and her colleagues surveyed 6,159 students at 32 colleges and universities across the United States. Here's what they found out:

- One in four women reported being raped or a victim of attempted rape.

- 84% of these women knew their attackers; 57% of sexual assaults occurred in a dating context.

- 12% of the men reported committing acts that met the legal definition of rape or attempted rape.

- 75% of the men and 55% of the women reported using alcohol/other drugs before the assault.

In another study, about 30% of men and women reported being "mildly buzzed" during sexual assault.

What's the Relationship between Sexual Assault and Alcohol?

- Many men's expectations are changed when they drink alcohol. Some men think that alcohol makes them more sexually aroused. (Think about ads for alcohol and what people are told they will feel.)

- Men may misperceive women's sexual intent. In comparison to women, men tend to interpret verbal and nonverbal behavior (including ambiguous cues) in a more sexualized fashion.

- Use of alcohol becomes a way for some men to justify sexual violence. Alcohol provides some guys with an excuse to "write off" or dismiss their behavior ("It wasn't me; it was the alcohol").

- Alcohol affects women's ability to send and receive cues about their sexual intent. The more intoxicated they become, the more their judgment and ability to think sharply become impaired, making it hard to "read" and quickly make sense of what's going on between women and men.

(p. 1 of 2; continued)

• • •

- Alcohol affects a woman's ability to resist sexual assault. It's hard for a woman to think quickly, get out of a sticky situation, or fight back when she's drunk or passed out.

- A lot of guys think women are "easier" and "looser" after drinking alcohol.

- Another problem is that women are at a disadvantage when drinking with men, because of differences in how women process alcohol. For example, men have five times more alcohol dehydrogenase (a stomach enzyme that helps metabolize alcohol) than women. Men also usually weigh more and have more bodily fluids; both of these factors help dilute the alcohol). By comparison, a woman gets a lot more drunk on the same amount of alcohol even when she weighs as much as a man. If a woman is matching drinks with a man, she may easily get twice as drunk as he does.

APPENDIX D

A Selection of Published and Unpublished Assessment Measures

COMPREHENSIVE EFFECTS OF ALCOHOL (CEA)

This questionnaire assesses two things:

1) what you would expect to happen if you were under the influence of alcohol, and
2) whether you think the effect is good or bad.

INSTRUCTIONS

A. Choose from "disagree to agree" depending on whether you expect the effect to happen to you *if you were under the influence of alcohol*. These effects will vary, depending on the amount of alcohol you typically consume. *Circle one answer for the first set of numbers after each statement.*

B. Choose from BAD TO GOOD depending on whether you think the particular effect is bad, neutral, good, etc. We want to know if you think a particular effect is bad or good, regardless of whether or not you expect it to happen to you. Circle only one answer for the last set of numbers after each statement.

Example: 1. I would be. . . . 1 2 3 4 This effect is 1 2 3 4 5

	1 = Disagree 2 = Slightly Disagree		1 = Bad 2 = Slightly Bad 3 = Neutral
IF I WERE UNDER THE INFLUENCE FROM DRINKING ALCOHOL:	3 = Slightly Agree 4 = Agree		4 = Slightly Good 5 = Good
1. I would be outgoing	1 2 3 4	This effect is	1 2 3 4 5
2. My senses would be dulled	1 2 3 4	This effect is	1 2 3 4 5
3. I would be humorous	1 2 3 4	This effect is	1 2 3 4 5
4. My problems would seem worse	1 2 3 4	This effect is	1 2 3 4 5
5. It would be easier to express my feelings	1 2 3 4	This effect is	1 2 3 4 5
6. My writing would be impaired	1 2 3 4	This effect is	1 2 3 4 5
7. I would feel sexy	1 2 3 4	This effect is	1 2 3 4 5
8. I would have difficulty thinking	1 2 3 4	This effect is	1 2 3 4 5
9. I would neglect my obligations	1 2 3 4	This effect is	1 2 3 4 5
10. I would be dominant	1 2 3 4	This effect is	1 2 3 4 5
11. My head would feel fuzzy	1 2 3 4	This effect is	1 2 3 4 5
12. I would enjoy sex more	1 2 3 4	This effect is	1 2 3 4 5

(p. 1 of 2; continued)

13. I would feel dizzy	1	2	3	4	This effect is	1	2	3	4	5
14. I would be friendly	1	2	3	4	This effect is	1	2	3	4	5
15. I would be clumsy	1	2	3	4	This effect is	1	2	3	4	5
16. It would be easier to act out my fantasies	1	2	3	4	This effect is	1	2	3	4	5
17. I would be loud, boisterous, or noisy	1	2	3	4	This effect is	1	2	3	4	5
18. I would feel peaceful	1	2	3	4	This effect is	1	2	3	4	5
19. I would be brave and daring	1	2	3	4	This effect is	1	2	3	4	5
20. I would feel unafraid	1	2	3	4	This effect is	1	2	3	4	5
21. I would feel creative	1	2	3	4	This effect is	1	2	3	4	5
22. I would be courageous	1	2	3	4	This effect is	1	2	3	4	5
23. I would feel shaky or jittery the next day	1	2	3	4	This effect is	1	2	3	4	5
24. I would feel energetic	1	2	3	4	This effect is	1	2	3	4	5
25. I would act aggressively	1	2	3	4	This effect is	1	2	3	4	5
26. My responses would be slow	1	2	3	4	This effect is	1	2	3	4	5
27. My body would be relaxed	1	2	3	4	This effect is	1	2	3	4	5
28. I would feel guilty	1	2	3	4	This effect is	1	2	3	4	5
29. I would feel calm	1	2	3	4	This effect is	1	2	3	4	5
30. I would feel moody	1	2	3	4	This effect is	1	2	3	4	5
31. It would be easier to talk to people	1	2	3	4	This effect is	1	2	3	4	5
32. I would be a better lover	1	2	3	4	This effect is	1	2	3	4	5
33. I would feel self-critical	1	2	3	4	This effect is	1	2	3	4	5
34. I would be talkative	1	2	3	4	This effect is	1	2	3	4	5
35. I would act tough	1	2	3	4	This effect is	1	2	3	4	5
36. I would take risks	1	2	3	4	This effect is	1	2	3	4	5
37. I would feel powerful	1	2	3	4	This effect is	1	2	3	4	5
38. I would act sociable	1	2	3	4	This effect is	1	2	3	4	5

DAILY DRINKING QUESTIONNAIRE (DDQ), Modified

INSTRUCTIONS

For each day of the week, fill in both the number of drinks consumed and the number of hours you typically drink.

Please be sure to fill out the information regarding your gender, weight, and height.

QUESTION 1

For the *past month*, please fill in a number for each day of the week indicating the *typical number of drinks* you usually consume on that day, and the *typical number of hours* you usually drink on that day.

Number of Drinks	Monday	Tuesday	Wednesday	Thursday	Friday	Saturday	Sunday
Number of Hours							

Weight _____ Gender _____ Height _____

QUESTION 2: RESIDENCE AND EMPLOYMENT

In the last quarter (or equivalent time period), please circle the most appropriate answers. Please choose one answer for each column. In responding to the question "Paid employment?", please circle the answer closest to the average number of hours you worked during that quarter.

Were you enrolled in college?   This college/university   Other college/university   No

Were you a Greek member?   Yes   No

Where did you live?   Greek house   Dorm   With parents   Apartment house   Other

Paid employment?   No   1/4 time   1/2 time   3/4 time   Full-time

FREQUENCY–QUANTITY QUESTIONNAIRE

Think of the occasion you drank the most this past month. How much did you drink?

1. No drinks
2. 1–2 drinks
3. 3–4 drinks
4. 5–6 drinks
5. 7–8 drinks
6. 9–10 drinks
7. 11–12 drinks
8. 13–14 drinks
9. 15–16 drinks
10. 17–18 drinks
11. 19 or more

On a given weekend evening, how much alcohol do you typically drink? Estimate for the past month.

1. No drinks
2. 1–2 drinks
3. 3–4 drinks
4. 5–6 drinks
5. 7–8 drinks
6. 9–10 drinks
7. 11–12 drinks
8. 13–14 drinks
9. 15–16 drinks
10. 17–18 drinks
11. 19 or more

How often in the past month did you drink alchol?

1. I do not drink at all.
2. About once a month.
3. Two to three times a month.
4. Three to four times a month.
5. Nearly every day.
6. Once a day or more.

DRINKING NORMS RATING FORM

INSTRUCTIONS
Please choose one answer for questions 1 and 2.

1. Dormitory/residence hall
2. Fraternity
3. Sorority
4. With Parents
5. Own residence

1. What type of residence do you currently live in? _____
2. What type of residence do you expect to live in next semester? _____

INSTRUCTIONS	A. HOW OFTEN THEY DRINK	B. HOW MUCH THEY DRINK ON A TYPICAL WEEKEND EVENING
We are interested in your estimates of (A) *how often* and (B) *how much* different types of people drink. For the following questions, please assume whenever possible that you are *rating a typical person of your same sex*. In each of the following situations, please enter the corresponding number, giving one answer for (A) (1–7), and one answer for (B) (1–6).	1. Less than once a month 2. About once a month 3. Two or three times a month 4. Once or twice a week 5. Three or four times a week 6. Nearly every day 7. Once a day	1. 0 drinks 2. 1–2 drinks 3. 3–4 drinks 4. 5–6 drinks 5. 7–8 drinks 6. More than 8 drinks
3. An average college-bound senior in high school		
4. An average university student		
5. An average college student residing in a fraternity		
6. An average college student residing in a sorority		
7. An average college student residing in a dormitory/residence hall		
8. An average college student residing with his/her parents		
9. An average college student residing in his/her own residence		
10. Your closest friends		

ALCOHOL PERCEIVED RISKS ASSESSMENT (APRA)

How likely are you to engage in the following activities *in the future but during your college career?*

INSTRUCTIONS

1. Choose from "extremely unlikely" to "extremely likely," depending on whether you feel you expect to experience this activity during the next 4 years. Choose only one number for each statement.

2. Circle the number that most closely indicates your likelihood to participate in this experience.

UNLIKELY						LIKELY	
Extremely	Moderate	Mild	Neither	Mild	Moderate	Extremely	
1	2	3	4	5	6	7	1. Drive after drinking.
1	2	3	4	5	6	7	2. Have a hangover.
1	2	3	4	5	6	7	3. Feel nauseated or vomit due to drinking.
1	2	3	4	5	6	7	4. Experience blackouts.
1	2	3	4	5	6	7	5. Physically injure self while drinking.
1	2	3	4	5	6	7	6. Develop tolerance to alcohol (need more alcohol for the same effect).
1	2	3	4	5	6	7	7. Miss class due to hangover.
1	2	3	4	5	6	7	8. Attend class after drinking.
1	2	3	4	5	6	7	9. Receive a lower grade due to drinking.
1	2	3	4	5	6	7	10. Be unable to complete assignments on time due to drinking.
1	2	3	4	5	6	7	11. Caused shame or embarrassment to someone due to drinking.
1	2	3	4	5	6	7	12. Argue, act bad, or do mean things after drinking.
1	2	3	4	5	6	7	13. Do things that result in negative reactions from others while drinking.
1	2	3	4	5	6	7	14. Spend a lot of time on activities focused on drinking.
1	2	3	4	5	6	7	15. Develop a drinking problem.
1	2	3	4	5	6	7	16. Become an alcoholic.

From *Brief Alcohol Screening and Intervention for College Students (BASICS): A Harm Reduction Approach* by Linda A. Dimeff, John S. Baer, Daniel R. Kivlahan, and G. Alan Marlatt. Copyright 1999 by The Guilford Press. Permission to photocopy this form is granted to purchasers of *BASICS* for personal use only (see copyright page for details).

BRIEF SEXUAL BEHAVIORS SURVEY (BSBS)

INSTRUCTIONS

1. Read each question carefully and the several possible answers before you make your choice. Answer the questions by choosing the *one* response that is the *most accurate, in your opinion.*

2. Take as much time as you need. Work carefully and try to finish as soon as possible.

Circle the PERCENTAGE that you think most accurately answers the following questions. Choose only one response for each question.

1. What proportion of people your age at the university do you think have sexual intercourse at least once a month?

0% 10% 20% 30% 40% 50% 60% 70% 80% 90% 100%

2. What proportion of your close friends have sexual intercourse at least once a month?

0% 10% 20% 30% 40% 50% 60% 70% 80% 90% 100%

Please choose only one answer for this question by circling your response below.

3. Thinking back to sexual partners you have had over the past 6 months, were they:
   A. All male
   B. Mostly male, some female
   C. More male than female
   D. Equal numbers of male and female
   E. More female than male
   F. Mostly female, some male
   G. All female

❑ 4. How many times have you had sexual intercourse (vaginal or anal) in the last 3 months?

❑ 5. With how many different people have you had sexual intercourse in the last 3 months?

When you had sexual intercourse in the last 3 months, how many times had you:

❑ 6. Been drinking alcohol?

❑ 7. Been using marijuana or hashish?

❑ 8. Been using other drugs?

Please describe:_____
_____
_____

❑ 9. Used a condom?

Think back to the *most recent time* you had sexual intercourse. Choose one answer for each question.

10. Did you consume alcohol?   A. Yes B. No

11. Did you use marijuana   A. Yes B. No
    or hashish?

Check the box that corresponds to the extent to which you see yourself at risk (0 = not at all; 5 = very much).

0 1 2 3 4 5   14. Thinking about your sexual activities, to what extent do you see yourself at risk in terms of AIDS?

(p. 1 of 2; continued)

12. Did you use other drugs?   A. Yes B. No

Please explain: _____

_____

_____

13. Did you use a condom?   A. Yes B. No

0 1 2 3 4 5 15. Thinking about your sexual activities, to what extent do you see you or your partner(s) at risk in terms of pregnancy?

Statements 16 and 17 are statements about sexual activity and alcohol. Please check the blank in the appropriate column that best describes your opinion. Please check only one answer for each statement.

Agree Strongly	Agree Somewhat	Can't Decide	Disagree Somewhat	Disagree Strongly	
					16. I don't always keep to the rules I make for myself about sex when I've been drinking.
					17. If I've been drinking, it's easier for me to raise the issue of condoms or other safer sex techniques before having sex.

Statements 18 and 19 are about alcohol effects. Please check the blank in the appropriate column that best describes your opinion. Please check only one answer for each statement

Not at All	A Little	Some	Very Much	
				18. When I drink enough alcohol to feel the effects, I have sex with people that I wouldn't have sex with when I was sober.
				19. When I drink enough alcohol to feel the effects, I am more likely to do something sexually that is risky.

References

Abbey, A. (1982). Sex differences in attributions for friendly behavior: Do males misperceive females' friendliness? *Journal of Personality and Social Psychology, 42,* 830–838.

Abbey, A. (1987). Misperceptions of friendly behavior as sexual interest: A survey of naturally occurring incidents. *Psychology of Women Quarterly, 11,* 173–194.

Abbey, A. (1991). Acquaintance rape and alcohol consumption on college campuses: How are they linked? *Journal of American College Health, 39,* 165–169.

Abbey, A., & Melby, C. (1986). The effects of nonverbal cues of gender differences in perceptions of sexual intent. *Sex Roles, 15,* 283–298.

Agostinelli, G., Brown, J. M., & Miller, W. R. (1995). Effects of normative feedback on consumption among heavy drinking college students. *Journal of Drug Education, 25*(1), 31–40.

Alden, L. E. (1988). Behavioral self-management controlled-drinking strategies in a context of secondary prevention. *Journal of Consulting and Clinical Psychology, 56,* 280–286.

Allen, J. P., Maisto, S. A., & Connors, G. J. (1995). Self-report screening tests for alcohol problems in primary care. *Archives of Internal Medicine, 155,* 1726–1730.

Alterman, A. I. (1988). Patterns of familial alcoholism, alcohol severity, and psychopathology. *Journal of Nervous and Mental Diseases, 176,* 167–175.

Alterman, A. I., Bridges, K. R., & Tarter, R. E. (1986). Drinking behavior of high risk college men: Contradictory preliminary findings. *Alcoholism: Clinical and Experimental Research, 10,* 305–310.

American Psychiatric Association. (1987). *Diagnostic and statistical manual of mental disorders* (3rd ed., rev.). Washington, DC: Author.

American Psychiatric Association. (1994). *Diagnostic and statistical manual of mental disorders* (4th ed.). Washington, DC: Author.

Anderson, D. S., & Milgram, G. G. (1996). *Promising practices sourcebook: Campus alcohol strategies.* Fairfax, VA: George Mason University.

Anderson, P., & Scott, E. (1992). The effect of general practitioner's advice to heavy drinking men. *British Journal of Addiction, 87,* 891–900.

Armor, D. J., Pollich, J. M., & Stambul, H. B. (1978). *Alcoholism and treatment.* New York: Wiley.

Babor, T. F. (1990). Brief intervention strategies for harmful drinkers: New directions for medical education. *Canadian Medical Association Journal, 143,* 1070–1076.

Babor, T. F., Bolinsky, Z. S., Meyer, R. E., Hesselbrock, M. M., Hofman, M., & Howard, T. (1992). Types of alcoholics: Concurrent and predictive validity of some common classification schemes. *British Journal of Addiction, 87,* 1415–1431.

Babor, T. F., Hofman, M., DelBoca, F. K., Hesselbrock, V. M., Meyer, R. E., Dolinsky, Z. S., & Rounsaville, B. (1992). Types of alcoholics: I. Evidence for an empirically derived typology based on indicators of vulnerability and severity. Archives of General Psychiatry, 49, 599–608.

• • •

Baer, J. S. (1993). Etiology and secondary prevention of alcohol problems with young adults. In J. S. Baer, G. A. Marlatt, & R. J. McMahon (Eds.), *Addictive behaviors across the lifespan: Prevention, treatment, and policy issues* (pp. 111–137). Newbury Park, CA: Sage.

Baer, J. S., & Carney, M. M. (1993). Biases in the perceptions of the consequences of alcohol use among college students. *Journal of Studies on Alcohol, 54,* 54–60.

Baer, J. S., Kivlahan, D., Fromme, K., & Marlatt, G. A. (1989). A comparison of three methods of secondary prevention of alcohol abuse with college students: Preliminary results. In T. Loberg, W. R. Miller, G. A. Marlatt, & P. E. Nathan, (Eds.), *Addictive behaviors: Prevention and early intervention* (pp. 157–171). Amsterdam: Swets & Zeitlinger.

Baer, J. S., Kivlahan, D. R., & Marlatt, G. A. (1995). High-risk drinking across the transition from high school to college. *Alcoholism: Clinical and Experimental Research, 19,* 54–61.

Baer, J. S., Marlatt, G. A., Kivlahan, D. R., Fromme, K., Larimer, M. E., & Williams, E. (1992). An experimental test of three methods of alcohol risk-reduction with young adults. *Journal of Consulting and Clinical Psychology, 60,* 974–979.

Baer, J. S., Stacy, A., & Larimer, M. (1991). Biases in the perception of drinking norms among college students. *Journal of Studies on Alcohol, 52,* 580–586.

Bandura, A. (1977). Self-efficacy: Toward a unifying theory of behavioral change. *Psychological Review, 84*(2), 191–215.

Barnes, G. M., Farrell, M. P., & Cairns, A. (1986). Parental socialization factors and adolescent drinking behaviors. *Journal of Marriage and the Family, 48,* 27–36.

Beadnell, B. A., Baker, S., Gordon, J. R., Roffman, R. A., & Craver, J. (1995, January). Risk reduction counseling groups with men who have sex with men and women who have sex with men. In J. R. Gordon (Chair), *Sexual health: A look at reducing sexual risk across a variety of populations.* Panel conducted at the Harm Reduction Conference, Seattle.

Berkowitz, A. D., & Perkins, H. W. (1986). Problem drinking among college students: A review of recent research. *Journal of American College Health, 35,* 21–28.

Bien, T. H., Miller, W. R., & Tonigan, J. S. (1993). Brief interventions for alcohol problems: A review. *Addiction, 88,* 315–335.

Bradley, K. A. (1992). Management of alcoholism in the primary care setting. *Western Journal of Medicine, 156,* 273–277.

Brehm, S. S., & Brehm, J. W. (1981). *Psychological reactance: A theory of freedom and control.* New York: Academic Press.

Brennan, A. F., Walfish, S., & AuBuchon, P. (1986). Alcohol use and abuse in college students: I. A review of individual and personality correlates. *International Journal of the Addictions, 21,* 449–474.

Brickman, P., Rabinowitz, V. C., Karnza, J., Coates, D., Cohn, E., & Kidder, L. (1983). Models of helping and coping. *American Psychologist, 37,* 368–384.

Brown, S. A., Christensen, B. A., & Goldman, M. S. (1987). The Alcohol Expectancies Questionnaire: An instrument for the assessment of adolescent and adult alcohol expectancies. *Journal of Studies on Alcohol, 48,* 483–491.

Brown, S. A., Craemer, V. A., & Stetson, B. A. (1987). Adolescent alcohol expectancies in relation to personal and parental drinking patterns. *Journal of Abnormal Psychology, 96,* 117–121.

Brown, S. A., Goldman, M. S., Inn, A., & Anderson, L. R. (1980). Expectations of reinforcement from alcohol: Their domain and relation to drinking patterns. *Journal of Consulting and Clinical Psychology, 48,* 419–426.

Bry, B., McKeon, P., & Padina, R. J. (1982). Extent of drug use as a function of number of risk factors. *Journal of Abnormal Psychology, 91,* 273–279.

Cadoret, R. J. (1990). Genetics of alcoholism. In R. L. Collins, K. E. Leonard, & J. S. Searles (Eds.), *Alcohol and the family* (pp. 39–78). New York: Guilford Press.

Cahalan, D., & Cisin, I. H. (1968). American drinking practices: Summary of finding from a national probability sample. *Quarterly Journal of Studies on Alcohol, 29,* 130–151.

Cahalan, D., Cisin, I. H., & Crossley, H. M. (1969). *American drinking practices.* New Brunswick, NJ: Rutgers Center of Alcohol Studies.

Campbell, K. E., Zobeck, T. S., & Bertolucci, D. (1995). *Trends in alcohol-related fatal traffic crashes, United States, 1977–1993* (Surveillance Report No. 34). Rockville, MD: U.S. Department of Health and Human Services.

Campbell, M. K., DeVellis, B. M., Strecher, V. J., Ammerman, A. S., DeVellis, R. F., & Sandler, R. S. (1994). Improving dietary behavior: The effectiveness of tailored messages in primary care settings. *American Journal of Public Health, 84,* 783–787.

Carskadon, M. A., & Dement, W. C. (1989). Normal sleep and its variations. In M. H. Kryger, T. Roth, & W. C. Dement (Eds.), *Principles and practice of sleep medicine.* Philadelphia: Saunders.

Christensen, A., & Jacobson, N. S. (1994). Who (or what) can do psychotherapy?: The status and challenge of nonprofessional therapies. *Psychological Science, 5,* 8–14.

Christensen, B. A., Goldman, M. S., & Brown, S. A. (1985). The differential development of adolescent alcohol expectancies may predict adult alcoholism. *Addictive Behaviors, 10,* 299–306.

Cohen, S. J., Stookey, G. K., Katz, B. P., Brook, C. A., & Smith, D. M. (1989). Encouraging primary care physicians to help smokers quit: A randomized, controlled trial. *Annals of Internal Medicine, 110,* 648–652.

Collins, R. L., Parks, G. A., & Marlatt, G. A. (1985). Social determinants of alcohol consumption: The effects of social interaction and model status on the self-administration of alcohol. *Journal of Consulting and Clinical Psychology, 53,* 189–200.

Curry, S. J., Kristal, A. R., & Bowen, D. J. (1992). An application of the stage model of behavior change to dietary fat reduction. *Health Education Research, 7,* 97–105.

Derogatis, L. R. (1977). *The SCL-90 manual: Vol. 1. Scoring, administration, and procedures.* Baltimore: Clinical Psychometric Research.

Derogatis, L. R., & Spencer, P. M. (1982). *The Brief Symptom Inventory (BSI) manual: Vol. 1. Administration, scoring, and procedures.* Baltimore: Johns Hopkins School of Medicine.

Dimeff, L. A. (1996). *Primary care providers' BASICS manual.* Unpublished manuscript.

Dimeff, L. A., Baer, J. S., & Marlatt, G. A. (1994). *Differential risks for college women drinkers.* Unpublished manuscript.

Dimeff, L. A., Kilmer, J., Baer, J. S., & Marlatt, G. A. (1995). Binge drinking in college [Letter, comment]. *Journal of the American Medical Association, 273,* 1903–1904.

Dimeff, L. A., & Marlatt, G. A. (1995). Relapse prevention. In R. Hester & W. R. Miller (Eds.), *Handbook of alcoholism treatment approaches: Effective alternatives* (2nd ed., pp. 176–194). Needham Heights, MA: Allyn & Bacon.

Donovan, C., & McEwan, R. (1995). A review of the literature examining the relationship between alcohol use and HIV-related sexual risk-taking in young people. *Addiction, 90*(3), 319–328.

Donovan, D. M. (1995). Assessments to aid in the treatment planning process. In J. P. Allen & M. Columbus (Eds.), *Assessing alcohol problems: A guide for clinicians and researchers* (NIAAA Treatment Handbook Series No. 4, DHHS Publication No. 95-3745). Washington, DC: U.S. Government Printing Office.

Donovan, D. M., Rohsenow, D. J., Schau, E. J., & O'Leary, M. R. (1977). Defensive styles in alcoholics and non-alcoholics. *Journal of Studies on Alcohol, 38,* 465–470.

Duthie, L. A., Baer, J. S., & Marlatt, G. A. (1991, November). *High risk status and personal risk perception for alcohol problems among college students.* Poster presented at the annual convention of the Association for Advancement of Behavior Therapy, New York.

• • •

Edwards, G., Orford, J., Egert, S., Guthrie, S., Hawker, A., Hensman, C., Mitcheson, M., Oppenheimer, E., & Taylor, C. (1977). Alcoholism: A controlled trial of "treatment" and "advice." *Journal of Studies on Alcohol, 38,* 1004–1031.

Engs, R. C., & Hanson, D. J. (1985). The drinking-patterns and problems of college students: 1983. *Journal of Alcohol and Drug Education, 31,* 65–82.

Engs, R. C., & Hanson, D. J. (1990). Gender differences in drinking patterns and problems among college students: A review of the literature. *Journal of Alcohol and Drug Education, 35,* 36–47.

Engs, R. C., Diebold, B. A., & Hanson, D. J. (1994). The drinking patterns and problems of a national sample of college students. *Journal of Alcohol and Drug Education, 41,* 13–33.

Erickson, P. G., Riley, P. G., Cheung, Y. W., & O'Hare, P. A. (1997). *Harm reduction: A new direction for drug policies and programs.* Toronto: University of Toronto Press.

Fillmore, K. M. (1988). *Alcohol use across the life course.* Toronto: Addiction Research Foundation.

Fingarette, H. (1988). *Heavy drinking: The myth of alcoholism as a disease.* Berkeley: University of California Press.

First, M. B., Spitzer, R. L., Gibbon, M., & Williams, J. B. W. (1995). *Structured Clinical Interview for DSM-IV Axis I Disorders—Patient Edition* (Version 2. 0). New York: Biometrics Research Department, New York State Psychiatric Institute.

Frezza, M., DiPadova, C., Pozzato, G., Terpin, M., Baraona, E., & Lieber, C. S. (1990). High blood alcohol levels in women: The role of decreased gastric alcohol dehydrogenase activity and first-pass metabolism. *New England Journal of Medicine, 322,* 95–99.

Fromme, K., Kivlahan, D. R., & Marlatt, G. A. (1986). Alcohol expectancies, risk identification, and secondary prevention with problem drinkers. *Advances in Behavior Research and Therapy, 8,* 237–251.

Fromme, K., Stroot, E. A., & Kaplan, D. (1993). Comprehensive Effects of Alcohol: Development and psychometric assessment of a new expectancy questionnaire. *Psychological Assessment, 5,* 19–26.

Gadaleto, A. F., & Anderson, D. S. (1984). Continued progress: The 1979, 1982, and 1985 college alcohol surveys. *Journal of College Student Personnel, 27*(6), 499–509.

Garner, D. M., Olmsted, M. P., Bohr, Y., & Garfinkel, P. E. (1982). The Eating Attitudes Test: Psychometric features and clinical correlates. *Psychological Medicine, 12,* 871–878.

Geller, E. S., & Kalsher, M. J. (1990). Environmental determinants of party drinking: Bartenders vs. self-service. *Environment and Behavior, 22,* 74–90.

Geller, E. S., Russ, N. W., & Altomari, M. G. (1986). Naturalistic observations of beer drinking among college students. *Journal of Applied Behavior Analysis, 19,* 391–396.

George, W. H., Cue, K. L., Lopez, P. A., Crowe-Leif, C. (1995). Self-reported alcohol expectancies and postdrinking sexual inference about women. *Journal of Applied Social Psychology, 25,* 164–186.

George, W. H., Gournic, S. J., & McAfee, M. P. (1988). Perceptions of post-drinking female sexuality: Effects of gender, beverage choice and drink payment. *Journal of Applied Social Psychology, 18,* 1295–1317.

George, W. H., & Marlatt, G. A. (1986). The effects of alcohol and anger on interest in violence, erotica, and deviance. *Journal of Abnormal Psychology, 95,* 150–158.

Gilpin, E. A., Pierce, J. P., Johnson, M., & Bal, D. (1993). Physician advice to quit smoking: Results from the 1990 California tobacco survey. *Journal of General Internal Medicine, 8,* 549–553.

Glasser, W. (1976). *Positive addiction.* New York: Harper & Row.

Golding, J. M., Siegel, J. M., Sorenson, S. B., Burnam, M. A., & Stein, C. H. (1989). Social support sources following sexual assault. *Journal of Community Psychology, 17,* 92–107.

Gordon, R. (1987). An operational classification of disease prevention. In J. A. Steinberg & M. M. Silverman (Eds.), *Preventing mental disorders: A research perspective* (DHHS Publication No. [ADM] 87-1492, pp. 20–26). Rockville, MD: National Institute of Mental Health.

Grant, B. F., Harford, T. C., & Grigson, M. B. (1988). Stability of alcohol consumption among youth: A national longitudinal survey. *Journal of Studies on Alcohol, 49,* 253–260.

Hall, S. M., Havassy, B. E., & Wasserman, D. A. (1990). Commitment to abstinence and acute stress in relapse to alcohol, opiates, and nicotine. *Journal of Consulting and Clinical Psychology, 58,* 175–181.

Harburg, E., Davis, D. R., & Caplan, R. (1982). Parent and offspring alcohol use: Imitative and aversive transmission. *Journal of Studies on Alcohol, 43,* 497–516.

Hay, W. M., & Nathan, P. E. (1982). *Clinical case studies in the behavioral treatment of alcoholism.* New York: Plenum Press.

Hays, R. D., & Ellickson, P. L. (1990). How generalizable are adolescents' beliefs about pro-drug pressures and resistance self-efficacy? *Journal of Applied Social Psychology, 20,* 321–340.

Heather, N. (1995). Brief intervention strategies . In R. Hester & W. R. Miller (Eds.), *Handbook of alcoholism treatment approaches: Effective alternatives* (2nd ed., pp. 105–122). Needham Heights, MA: Allyn & Bacon.

Hester, R. K. (1995). Behavioral self-control training. In R. K. Hester & W. R. Miller (Eds.), *Handbook of alcoholism treatment approaches: Effective alternatives* (2nd ed., pp. 148–159). Needham Heights, MA: Allyn & Bacon.

Hester, R. K., & Miller, W. R. (Eds.). (1995). *Handbook of alcoholism treatment approaches: Effective alternatives.* Needham Heights, MA: Allyn & Bacon.

Hull, J. G., & Bond, C. F. (1986). Social and behavioral consequences of alcohol consumption and expectancy: A meta-analysis. *Psychological Bulletin, 99,* 347–360.

Hurlbut, S. C., & Sher, K. J. (1992). Assessing alcohol problems in college students. *Journal of American College Health, 41,* 49–58.

Institute of Medicine. (1990). *Broadening the base of treatment for alcohol problems.* Washington, DC: National Academy Press.

Institute of Medicine. (1995). *Weighing the options: Criteria for evaluating weight-management programs.* Washington, DC: National Academy Press.

Jacob, T., & Leonard, K. (1991). Experimental drinking procedures in the study of alcoholics and their families: A consideration of ethical issues. *Journal of Consulting and Clinical Psychology, 59,* 249–255.

Jellinek, E. M. (1960). *The disease model of alcoholism.* Highland Park, NJ: Hillhouse Press.

Jessor, R. (1991). Risk behavior in adolescence: A psychosocial framework for understanding and action. *Journal of Adolescent Health, 12,* 587–605.

Jessor, R. (1993). Successful adolescent development among youth in high-risk settings. *American Psychologist, 48,* 117–126.

Jessor, R., Donovan, J. E., & Costa, F. M. (1991). *Beyond adolescence: Problem behavior and young adult development.* New York: Cambridge University Press.

Jessor, R., & Jessor, S. L. (1977). *Problem behavior and psychosocial development: A longitudinal study of youth.* New York: Academic Press.

Johnston, L. D., O'Malley, P. M., & Bachman, J. G. (1992). *Smoking, drinking, and illicit drug use among American secondary school students, college students, and young adults, 1975–1991.* Rockville, MD: U.S. Department of Health and Human Services.

Johnston, L. D., O'Malley, P. M., & Bachman, J. G. (1996). *National survey results on drug use from the Monitoring the Future Study, 1975–1994: Vol. 2. College students and young adults.* Rockville, MD: U.S. Department of Health and Human Services, Public Health Service, National Institutes of Health.

Jones, B. M., & Jones, M. K. (1976). Male and female intoxication levels for three alcohol doses, or do women really get higher than men? A brief communication. *Alcohol Technical Reports, 5,* 11–14.

Jones-Saumty, D. J., & Zeiner, A. R. (1985). Psychological correlates of drinking behavior in social drinker college students. *Alcoholism: Clinical and Experimental Research, 9,* 158–163.

Kadden, R., Carroll, K., Donovan, D., Cooney, N., Monti, P., Abrams, D., Litt, M., & Hester, R. (1994). *Cognitive-behavioral coping skills therapy manual: A clinical research guide for therapists treating individuals with alcohol abuse and dependence* (NIAAA Project MATCH Monograph Series, Volume 3). Rockville, MD: U.S. Department of Health and Human Services.

Kandel, D. B., & Andrews, K. (1987). Processes of adolescent socialization by parents and peers. *International Journal of the Addictions, 22,* 319–342.

Kanin, E. J. (1985). Date rapists: Differential sexual socialization and reactive deprivation. *Archives of Sexual Behavior, 14,* 218–232.

Kay, D. C., & Samiuddin, Z. (1988). Sleep disorders associated with drug abuse and drugs of abuse. In R. L. Williams, I. Karacan, & C. A. Moore (Eds.), *Sleep disorders: Diagnosis and treatment* (pp. 315–371). New York: Wiley.

Keller, D. S., Bennett, M. E., McCrady, B. S., Paulus, M. D., & Frankenstein, W. (1994). Treating college substance abusers: The New Jersey collegiate substance abuse program. *Journal of Substance Abuse Treatment, 11*(6), 569–581.

Kilmer, J. R., Larimer, M. E., Baer, J. S., Parks, G. A., Dimeff, L. A., & Marlatt, G. A. (1995). *Predictors of fraternity and sorority members to constraints on drinking.* Manuscript submitted for publication.

Kilmer, J., Larimer, M., & Marlatt, G. A. (1997). *An analysis of drinking behavior, house reputation, and situation-specific expectancies among fraternity and sorority members.* Manuscript submitted for publication.

King, C. A., Ghaziuddin, N., McGovern, L., & Brand, E. (1996). Predictors of comorbid alcohol and substance abuse in depressed adolescents. *Journal of the American Academy of Child and Adolescent Psychiatry, 35*(6), 743–751.

Kishline, A. (1994). *Moderate drinking: The new option for problem drinkers.* San Francisco: See Sharp Press.

Kivlahan, D. R., Marlatt, G. A., Fromme, K., Coppel, D. B., & Williams, E. (1990). Secondary prevention with college drinkers: Evaluation of an alcohol skills training program. *Journal of Consulting and Clinical Psychology, 58,* 805–810.

Klatsky, A. L., & Armstrong, M. A. (1993). Alcohol use, other traits, and risk of unnatural death: A prospective study. *Alcoholism: Clinical and Experimental Research, 17,* 1156–1162.

Klatsky, A. L., Friedman, G. D., & Giegelaub, A. B. (1981). Alcohol and mortality: A ten-year Kaiser-Permanente experience. *Annals of Internal Medicine, 95,* 139–145.

Koss, M. P., & Dinero, T. E. (1989). Discriminant analysis of risk factors for sexual victimization among a national sample of college women. *Journal of Consulting and Clinical Psychology, 57,* 242–250.

Koss, M. P., & Gidycz, C. A. (1985). Sexual Experiences Survey: Reliability and validity. *Journal of Consulting and Clinical Psychology, 53,* 422–423.

Koss, M. P., Gidycz, C. A., & Wisniewski, N. (1987). The scope of rape: Incidence and prevalence of sexual aggression and victimization in a national sample of higher education students. *Journal of Clinical and Consulting Psychology, 55,* 162–170.

Koss, M. P., & Oros, C. J. (1982). The Sexual Experiences Survey: A research instrument investigating sexual aggression and victimization. *Journal of Consulting and Clinical Psychology, 50,* 455–457.

Kottke, T. E., Battista, R. N., DeFriese, G. H., & Brekke, M. L. (1988). Attributes of successful smoking cessation interventions in medical practice: A meta-analysis of 39 controlled trials. *Journal of the American Medical Association, 259,* 2883–2889.

Krahn, D. D. (1991). The relationship of eating disorders and substance abuse. *Journal of Substance Abuse, 3,* 239–253.

Lall, R., & Schandler, S. L. (1991). Michigan Alcohol Screening Test (MAST) scores and academic performance in college students. *College Student Journal, 25*(2), 245–251.

Larimer, M. E. (1992). *Alcohol abuse and the Greek system: An exploration of fraternity and sorority drinking.* Unpublished doctoral dissertation, University of Washington.

Leigh, B. C. (1987). Evaluations of alcohol expectancies: Do they add to prediction of drinking patterns? *Psychology of Addictive Behaviors, 1,* 135–139.

Leigh, B. C. (1989). Attitudes and expectancies as predictors of drinking habits: A comparison of three scales. *Journal of Studies on Alcohol, 50,* 432–440.

Linehan, M. M. (1993). *Cognitive-behavioral treatment of borderline personality disorder.* New York: Guilford Press.

Litt, M. D., Babor, T. F., DelBoca, F. K., Kadden, R. M., & Cooney, N. L. (1992). Types of alcoholics: II. Application of an empirically derived typology to treatment matching. *Archives of General Psychiatry, 49,* 609–614.

Lowell, N. (1993, December). *University life and substance abuse: 1993 survey* (Report No. 93-4). University of Washington, Office of Educational Assessment.

Luce, K. H., DuBoise, H. M., Dimeff, L. A., Larimer, M. E., & Marlatt, G. A. (1993). *Exploring the relationship between problematic eating and drinking behaviors among sorority women.* Unpublished manuscript.

Mace, F. C., & Kratochwill, T. R. (1985). Theories of reactivity in self-monitoring: A comparison of cognitive-behavioral and operant models. *Behavior Modification, 9,* 323–343.

Manley, M. W., Epps, R. P., & Glynn, T. J. (1992). The clinician's role in promoting smoking cessation among clinic patients. *Medical Clinics of North America, 76,* 477–494.

Mann, L. M., Cassin, L., & Sher, K. J. (1987). Alcohol expectancies and the risk of alcoholism. *Journal of Consulting and Clinical Psychology, 55,* 411–417.

Mann, R. E., Sobell, L. C., Sobell, L. C., & Pavan, D. (1985). Reliability of a Family Tree Questionnaire for assessing family history of alcohol problems. *Drug and Alcohol Dependence, 15,* 61–67.

Marlatt, G. A. (1987). Alcohol, the magic elixir: Stress, expectancy, and the transformation of emotional states. In E. Gottheil, K. A. Druly, S. Pashko, & S. P. Weinstein (Eds.), *Stress and addiction* (pp. 302–322). New York: Brunner/Mazel.

Marlatt, G. A. (Ed.). (1998a). *Harm reduction: Pragmatic strategies for managing high-risk behaviors.* New York: Guilford Press.

Marlatt, G. A. (1998b). Screening and brief intervention for high-risk college student drinkers: Results from a two-year follow-up assessment. *Journal of Consulting and Clinical Psychology, 66,* 604–615.

Marlatt, G. A., Baer, J. S., Kivlahan, D. R., Dimeff, L. A., Larimer, M. E., Quigley, L. A., Somers, J. M., & Williams, E. (1998). Harm reduction for alcohol problems: Early intervention reduces drinking risks in college students. *Journal of Consulting and Clinical Psychology, 66,* 604–615.

Marlatt, G. A., Baer, J. S., & Larimer, M. (1995). Preventing alcohol abuse in college students: A harm-reduction approach. In G. M. Boyd, J. Howard, & R. A. Zucker (Eds.), *Alcohol problems among adolescents: Current directions in prevention research* (pp. 147–172). Hillsdale, NJ: Erlbaum.

Marlatt, G. A., & George, W. H. (1984). Relapse prevention: Introduction and overview of the model. *British Journal of Addiction, 79,* 261–273.

Marlatt, G. A., & Gordon, J. R. (1980). Determinants of relapse: Implications for the maintenance of behavior change. In P. O. Davidson & S. M. Davidson (Eds.), *Behavioral medicine: Changing lifestyles* (pp. 410–452). New York: Brunner/Mazel.

Marlatt, G. A., & Gordon, J. R. (Eds.). (1985). *Relapse prevention: Maintenance strategies in the treatment of addictive behaviors.* New York: Guilford Press.

Marlatt, G. A., Larimer, M. E., Baer, J. S., & Quigley, L. A. (1993). Harm reduction for alcohol problems: Moving beyond the controlled drinking controvery. *Behavior Therapy, 24,* 461–503.

Marlatt, G. A., & Nathan, P. E. (Eds.). (1978). *Behavioral approaches to alcoholism.* New Brunswick, NJ: Rutgers Center of Alcohol Studies.

Marlatt, G. A., & Rohsenow, D. R. (1980). Cognitive processes in alcohol use: Expectancy and the balanced placebo design. In N. K. Mello (Ed.), *Advances in substance abuse* (Vol. 1, pp. 159–199). Greenwich, CT: JAI Press.

Marlatt, G. A., & Tapert, S. F. (1993). Harm reduction: Reducing the risks of addictive behaviors. In J. S. Baer, G. A. Marlatt, & R. J. McMahon (Eds.), *Addictive behaviors across the lifespan: Prevention, treatment, and policy issues* (pp. 243–273). Newbury Park, CA: Sage.

Matthews, D. B., & Miller, W. R. (1979). Estimating blood alcohol concentration: Two computer programs and their application in treatment and research. *Addictive Behaviors, 4,* 55–60.

Mattson, M. E., & Allen, J. P. (1991). Research on matching alcoholic patients to treatments: Findings, issues, and implications. *Journal of Addictive Diseases, 11,* 33–49.

McConnaughy, E. A., Prochaska, J. O., & Velicer, W. F. (1983). Stages of change in psychotherapy: Measurement and sample profiles. *Psychotherapy: Theory, Research, and Practice, 20,* 368–375.

McLellan, A. T., Kushner, H., Metzger, D., Peters, F., et al. (1992). The fifth edition of the Addiction Severity Index. *Journal of Substance Abuse Treatment, 9,* 199–213.

McLellan, A. T., Luborsky, L., O'Brien, C. P., & Woody, G. E. (1980). An improved diagnostic instrument for substance abuse patients: The Addiction Severity Index. *Journal of Nervous and Mental Disease, 168,* 26–33.

McPhee, S. J., Bird, J. A., Rordham, D., Rodnick, J. E., & Osborn, E. H. (1991). Promoting cancer prevention activities by primary care physicians. *Journal of the American Medical Association, 266,* 538–544.

Meilman, P. W., von Hippel, F. A., & Gaylor, M. S. (1991). Self-induced vomiting in college women: Its relation to eating, alcohol use, and Greek life. *Journal of American College Health, 40,* 39–41.

Mercer, D., & Woody, G. (1992). *Addiction counseling.* Unpublished manuscript.

Milam, J. R., & Ketcham, K. (1981). *Under the influence: A guide to the myths and realities of alcoholism.* Seattle, WA: Madrona Press.

Miller, P. M., & Nirenberg, T. D. (Eds.). (1984). *Prevention of alcohol abuse.* New York: Plenum Press.

Miller, W. R. (1976). Alcoholism scales and objective assessment methods: A review. *Psychological Bulletin, 83,* 649–674.

Miller, W. R. (1985). Motivation for treatment: A review with special emphasis on alcoholism. *Psychological Bulletin, 98,* 84–107.

Miller, W. R., Brown, J. M., Simpson, T. L., Handmaker, N. S., Bien, T. H., Luckie, L. F., Montgomery, H. A., Hester, R. K., & Tonigan, J. S. (1995). What works?: A methodological analysis of the alcohol treatment outcome literature. In R. Hester & W. R. Miller (Eds.), *Handbook of alcoholism treatment approaches: Effective alternatives* (2nd ed., pp. 12–44). Needham Heights, MA: Allyn & Bacon.

Miller, W. R., & Marlatt, G. A. (1984). *Brief Drinker Profile.* Odessa, FL: Psychological Assessment Resources.

Miller, W. R., & Munoz, R. F. (1982). *How to control your drinking: A practical guide to responsible drinking* (rev. ed.). Albuquerque: University of New Mexico Press.

Miller, W. R., & Rollnick, S. (1991). *Motivational interviewing: Preparing people for change.* New York: Guilford Press.

Miller, W. R., & Sovereign, R. G. (1989). The check-up: A model for early intervention in addictive behaviors. In T. Loberg, W. R. Miller, P. E. Nathan, & G. A. Marlatt (Eds.), *Addictive behaviors: Prevention and early intervention* (pp. 219–231). Amsterdam: Swets & Zeitlinger.

Miller, W. R., Sovereign, R. G., & Krege, B. (1988). Motivational interviewing with problem drinkers: II. The drinker's check-up as a preventive intervention. *Behavioural Psychotherapy, 16,* 251–268.

Miller, W. R., Tonigan, J. S., & Longabaugh, R. (1995). *The Drinker Inventory of Consequences (DrInC) of Alcohol Abuse: Test manual* (NIAAA Project MATCH Monograph No. 4, DHHS Publication No. 95-3911). Rockville, MD: National Institute of Alcohol Abuse and Alcoholism.

Miller, W. R., Zweben, A., DiClemente, C. C., & Rychtarik, R. G. (1992). *Motivational enhancement therapy manual.* Washington, DC: U.S. Government Printing Office.

Mitchell, J. E., Hatsukami, D., Eckert, E. D., & Pyle, R. L. (1985). Characteristics of 275 patients with bulimia. *American Journal of Psychiatry, 142,* 482–485.

Mooney, D. K., Fromme, K., Kivlahan, D. R., & Marlatt, G. A. (1987). Correlates of alcohol consumption: Sex, age, and expectancies relate differentially to quantity and frequency. *Addictive Behaviors, 12,* 235–240.

Mougin, F., Davenne, D., Simon, R. M. L., Renaud, A., Garnier, A., & Magnin, P. (1989). Disturbance of sports performance after partial deprivation. *Comptes Rendus des Séances de la Société de Biologie et de ses Filiales, 183,* 461–466.

Muehlenhard, C. L., & Linton, M. A. (1987). Date rape and sexual aggression in dating situations: Incidence and risk factors. *Journal of Counseling Psychology, 34,* 186–196.

National Highway Traffic Safety Administration. (1994). *Traffic safety facts 1993: A compilation of motor vehicle crash data from the Fatal Accident Reporting System and the General Estimates System.* Washington, DC: Author.

National Institute on Alcohol Abuse and Alcoholism (NIAAA). (1984). *Report of the 1983 Prevention Planning Panel.* Rockville, MD: U.S. Department of Health and Human Services.

National Institute on Alcohol Abuse and Alcoholism (NIAAA). (1992). Moderate drinking. *Alcohol Alert, 16,* 1.

National Institute on Alcohol Abuse and Alcoholism (NIAAA). (1993). *Eighth special report to the U. S. Congress on alcohol and health.* Rockville, MD: U.S. Department of Health and Human Services.

National Institute on Alcohol Abuse and Alcoholism (NIAAA). (1995). *Assessing alcohol problems.* Rockville, MD: U.S. Department of Health and Human Services.

Norris, J., Nurius, P. S., & Dimeff, L. A. (1996). Through her eyes: Perception of and resistance to acquaintance. *Psychology of Women Quarterly, 20*(1), 123–145.

Nowinski, J., Baker, S., & Carroll, K. (1994). *Twelve Step facilitation therapy manual: A clinical research guide for therapists treating individuals with alcohol abuse and alcohol dependence* (NIAAA Project MATCH Monograph Series, Vol. 1). Rockville, MD: U.S. Department of Health and Human Services.

O'Hare, T. M. (1990). Drinking in college: Consumption patterns, problems, sex differences and legal drinking age. *Journal of Studies on Alcohol, 51*(6), 536–541.

Ockene, J. K. (1987). Physician-delivered interventions for smoking cessation: Strategies for increasing effectiveness. *Preventive Medicine, 16,* 723–737.

Orford, J., Oppenheimer, E., & Edwards, G. (1976). Abstinence or control: The outcome for excessive drinkers two years after consultation. *Behaviour Research and Therapy, 14*(6), 409–418.

Pederson, L. L. (1982). Compliance with physician advice to quit smoking: A review of the literature. *Preventive Medicine, 11,* 71–84.

Perkins, H. W. (1992). Gender patterns in consequences of collegiate alcohol abuse: A 10-year study of trends in an undergraduate population. *Journal of Studies on Alcohol, 53,* 458–462.

Peveler, R., & Fairburn, C. (1990). Eating disorders in women who abuse alcohol. *British Journal of Addiction, 85,* 1633–1638.

Presley, C. A., Meilman, P. W., & Lyerla, R. (1994). Development of the Core Alcohol and Drug

Survey: initial findings and future directions. *Journal of American College Health, 42*(6), 248–255.

Presley, C. A., Meilman, P. W., & Lyerla, R. (1995). *Alcohol and drugs on American college campuses: Vol. 2. Use, consequences, and perceptions of the campus environment.* Carbondale: Southern Illinois University.

Prochaska, J. O., & DiClemente, C. C. (1984). *The transtheoretical approach: Crossing traditional boundaries of therapy.* Homewood, IL: Dow Jones/Irwin.

Prochaska, J. O., & DiClemente, C. C. (1986). Toward a comprehensive model of change. In W. R. Miller & N. Heather (Eds.), *Treating addictive behaviors: Processes of change* (pp. 3–27). New York: Plenum Press.

Prochaska, J. O., DiClemente, C. C., & Norcross, C. (1992). In search of how people change: Applications to addictive behaviors. *American Psychologist, 47,* 1102–1114.

Radomski, M. W., Hart, L. E., Goodman, J. M., & Plyley, M. J. (1992). Aerobic fitness and hormonal responses to prolonged sleep deprivation and sustained mental work. *Aviation, Space and Environmental Medicine, 63,* 101–106.

Rand, C. S. W., & Kuldau, J. M. (1992). Epidemiology of bulimia and symptoms in a general population: Sex, age, race, and socioeconomic status. *International Journal of Eating Disorders, 11,* 37–44.

Rand, C. S. W., Lawlor, B. A., & Kuldau, J. M. (1986). Patterns of food and alcohol consumption in a group of bulimic women. *Bulletin of the Society of Psychologists in Addictive Behaviors, 5,* 95–104.

Riley, D. (1994). *The harm reduction model: Pragmatic approaches to drug use from the area between intolerance and neglect.* Ottawa: Canadian Centre on Substance Abuse.

Rohsenow, D. J., & Marlatt, G. A. (1981). The balanced placebo design: Methodological considerations. *Addictive Behaviors, 6,* 107–122.

Rollnick, S., Heather, N., & Bell, A. (1992). Negotiating behaviour change in medical settings: The development of brief motivational interviewing. *Journal of Mental Health, 1,* 25–37.

Rollnick, S., Heather, N., Gold, R., & Hall, W. (1992). Development of a short "Readiness to Change Questionnaire" for use in brief, opportunistic interventions among excessive drinkers. *British Journal of Addictions, 87,* 743–754.

Saltz, R., & Elandt, D. (1986). College student drinking studies 1976–1985. *Contemporary Drug Problems, 13,* 117–159.

Sanchez-Craig, M., Annis, H. M., Bornet, A. R., & MacDonald, K. R. (1984). Random assignment to abstinence and controlled drinking: Evaluation of a cognitive-behavioral program for problem drinkers. *Journal of Consulting and Clinical Psychology, 52,* 390–403.

Sarason, I. G., Johnson, J. H., & Siegel, J. M. (1978). Assessing the impact of life changes: Development of the Life Experiences Survey. *Journal of Consulting and Clinical Psychology, 46,* 932–946.

Saunders, J. B., & Aasland, O. G. (Eds.). (1987). *WHO collaborative project on identification and treatment of persons with harmful alcohol consumption: Report on phase I development of a screening instrument.* Geneva: World Health Organization.

Schuckit, M. A. (1991). A longitudinal study of children of alcoholics. In M. Galanter (Ed.), *Recent developments in alcoholism* (Vol. 9, pp. 5–19). New York: Plenum Press.

Searles, J. S. (1990). The contribution of genetic factors to the development of alcoholism: A critical review. In R. L. Collins, K. E. Leonard, & J. S. Searles (Eds.), *Alcohol and the family* (pp. 3–38). New York: Guilford Press.

Selzer, M., Vinokur, A., & van Rooijen, L. A. (1976). A self-administered Short Michigan Alcoholism Screening Test (SMAST). *Journal of Studies on Alcohol, 36,* 117–126.

Shedler, J., & Block, J. (1990). Adolescent drug use and psychological health: A longitudinal inquiry. *American Psychologist, 45,* 612–630.

Sher, K. J., & Descutner, C. (1986). Reports of paternal alcoholism: Reliability across siblings. *Addictive Behaviors, 11,* 25–30.

Sher, K. J., Walitzer, K. S., Wood, P. K., & Brent, E. E. (1991). Characteristics of children of alcoholics: Putative risk factors, substance use and abuse, and psychopathology. *Journal of Abnormal Psychology, 100,* 427–448.

Skinner, C. S., Strecher, V. J., & Hospers, H. (1994). Physicians' recommendations for mammography: Do tailored messages make a difference? *American Journal of Public Health, 84,* 12–13.

Skinner, H. A., & Allen, B. A. (1983). Does the computer make a difference?: Computerized versus face-to-face versus self-report assessment of alcohol, drug, and tobacco use. *Journal of Consulting and Clinical Psychology, 51,* 267–275.

Skinner, H. A., & Horn, J. L. (1984). *Alcohol Dependence Scale (ADS) user's guide.* Toronto: Addiction Research Foundation.

Sobell, M. B., & Sobell, L. C. (1993). Treatment for problem drinkers: A public health priority. In J. S. Baer, G. A. Marlatt, & R. J. McMahon (Eds.), *Addictive behaviors across the lifespan: Prevention, treatment, and policy issues* (pp. 138–157). Newbury Park, CA: Sage.

Solomon, R. L. (1980). The opponent-process theory of acquired motivation: The cost of pleasure and the benefits of pain. *American Psychologist, 35,* 691–712.

Solomon, R. L., & Corbit, J. D. (1974). An opponent-process theory of acquired motivation: I. Temporal dynamics of affect. *Psychological Review, 81,* 119–145.

Somers, J. M., Baer, J. S., & Marlatt, G. A. (1991, March). *Student drinking across the transition from high school to university and the role of residence type.* Poster presented at the Banff International Conference on Behavioural Science, Banff, Alberta, Canada.

Southwick, L., Steele, C., Marlatt, G. A., & Lindell, M. (1981). Alcohol-related expectancies: Defined by phase of intoxication and drinking experience. *Journal of Consulting and Clinical Psychology, 49,* 713–721.

Stacy, A. W., Sussman, S., Dent, C. W., Burton, D., & Flay, B. R. (1992). Moderators of peer social influence in adolescent smoking. *Personality and Social Psychology Bulletin, 18,* 163–172.

Stacy, A. W., Widaman, K. F., & Marlatt, G. A. (1990). Expectancy models of alcohol use. *Journal of Personality and Social Psychology, 58,* 918–928.

Stangler, R. S., & Printz, A. M. (1980). DSM-III: Psychiatric diagnosis in a university population. *American Journal of Psychiatry, 137,* 937–940.

Steele, C. M., & Josephs, R. A. (1990). Alcohol myopia: Its prized and dangerous effects. *American Psychologist, 45,* 921–933.

Straus, R., & Bacon, S. D. (1953). *Drinking in college.* New Haven, CT: Yale University Press.

Strecher, V. J., Kobrin, S. C., Kreuter, M. W., Roodhouse, K., & Farrell, D. (1994). Opportunities for alcohol screening and counseling in primary care. *Journal of Family Practice, 39,* 26–32.

Streissguth, A. P. (1983). Alcohol and pregnancy: An overview and an update. *Substance and Alcohol Actions/Misuse, 4,* 149–173.

Streissguth, A. P., Barr, H. M., Sampson, P. D., & Bookstein, F. L. (1994). Prenatal alcohol and offspring development: The first fourteen years. *Drug and Alcohol Dependence, 36,* 89–99.

Strunin, L., & Hingson, R. (1992). Alcohol, drugs, and adolescent sexual behavior. *International Journal of the Addictions, 27*(2), 129–146.

Szmukler, G. I., & Tantam, D. (1984). Anorexia nervosa: Starvation dependence. *British Journal of Medical Psychology, 57,* 303–310.

Tarter, R. E. (1991). Developmental behavior-genetic perspectives of alcoholism etiology. In M. Galanter (Ed.), *Recent developments in alcoholism* (Vol. 9, pp. 71–85). New York: Plenum Press.

Tarter, R. E., Arria, A. M., Moss, H., Edwards, N. J., & Van Thiel, D. H. (1987). DSM-III criteria for alcohol abuse: Associations with alcohol consumption behavior. *Alcoholism: Clinical and Experimental Research, 11*(6), 541–543.

Thompson, R. S., Michnich, M. E., Friedlander, L., Gilson, B., Grothaus, L. C., & Stoner, B. (1988).

Effectiveness of smoking cessation interventions integrated into primary care practice. *Medical Care, 26,* 62–76.

Tonigan, J. S., & Miller, W. R. (1993). Assessment and validation of the Drinker Inventory of Consequences (DrInC): A multi-site outpatient and aftercare clinical sample of problem drinkers. *Alcoholism: Clinical and Experimental Research, 17,* 513. (Abstract)

Tricker, R., & Cook, D. L. (1989). The current status of drug intervention & prevention in college athletic programs. *Journal of Alcohol and Drug Education, 34*(2), 38–45.

U.S. Department of Health and Human Services. (1993). *Eighth Special Report to the U.S. Congress on Alcohol and Health.* Alexandria, VA: EEI.

VanHelder, T., & Radomski, M. W. (1989). Sleep deprivation and the effect on exercise performance. *Sports Medicine, 7,* 235–247.

Vannicelli, M. (1989). *Group psychotherapy with adult children of alcoholics: Treatment techniques and countertransference considerations.* New York: Guilford Press.

Vannicelli, M. (1992). *Removing the roadblocks: Group psychotherapy with substance abusers and family members.* New York: Guilford Press.

Walfish, S., Wentz, D., Benzing, P., Brennan, F., & Champ, S. (1981). Alcohol abuse on a college campus: A needs assessment. *Evaluation and Program Planning, 4,* 163–168.

Wallace, P., Cutler, S., & Haines, A. (1988). Randomised controlled trial of general practitioner interventions in patients with excessive alcohol consumption. *British Medical Journal, 297,* 663–668.

Wang, T. H., & Katzev, R. D. (1990). Group commitment and resource conservation: Two field experiments on promoting recycling. *Journal of Applied Social Psychology, 20,* 265–275.

Watson, D. L., & Tharp, R. G. (1993). *Self-directed behavior: Self-modification for personal adjustment.* Pacific Grove, CA: Brooks/Cole.

Wechsler, H., Davenport, A., Dowdall, G., & Moeykens, B. (1994). Health and behavioral consequences of binge drinking in college: A national survey of students at 140 campuses. *Journal of the American Medical Association, 272,* 1672–1677.

Wechsler, H., & Isaac, N. (1992). "Binge" drinkers at Massachusetts colleges: Prevalence, drinking style, time trends, and associated problems. *Journal of the American Medical Association, 267,* 2929–2931.

Wechsler, H., Isaac, N. E., Grodstein, F., & Sellers, D. E. (1994). Continuation and initiation of alcohol use from the first to the second year of college. *Journal of Studies on Alcohol, 55,* 41–45.

White, H. R., & Labouvie, E. W. (1989). Towards the assessment of adolescent problem drinking. *Journal of Studies on Alcohol, 50,* 30–37.

Williams, I. M. (Ed.). (1982). *The American Heritage dictionary.* Boston: Houghton Mifflin.

Wilson, D. M. C., Lindsay, E. A., Best, J. A., Gilbert, J. R., Willms, D. G., & Singer, J. (1987). A smoking cessation intervention for family physicians. *Canadian Medical Association Journal, 137,* 613–619.

World Health Organization (WHO) Brief Intervention Study Group. (1996). A cross-national trial of brief interventions with heavy drinkers. *American Journal of Public Health, 86,* 948–955.

Yeary, J. R., & Heck, C. L. (1989). Dual diagnosis: Eating disorders and psychoactive substance dependence. *Journal of Psychoactive Drugs, 19,* 239–349.

Zucker, R. A., & Fitzgerald, H. E. (1991). Early developmental factors and risk for alcohol problems. *Alcohol Health and Research World, 15*(1), 18–24.

Zucker, R. A., Fitzgerald, H. E., & Moses, H. D. (1995). Emergence of alcohol problems and the several alcoholisms: A developmental perspective of etiological theory and life course trajectory. In D. Cicchetti & D. J. Cohen (Eds.), *Developmental psychopathology* (Vol. 2, pp. 677–711). New York: Wiley.

Index